the APPALACHIAN *trail* HIKER

For our daughter, Griffin.

Published by Menasha Ridge Press

Distributed by The Globe Pequot Press

Manufactured in Canada

Fourth edition, first printing

Library of Congress Cataloging-in-Publication Data

Logue, Victoria, 1961–

Appalachian Trail Hiker: formerly The Appalachian Trail Backpacker: trail-proven advice for A.T. hikes of any length/ Victoria and Frank Logue.

p. cm.

Rev. ed. of: The Appalachian Trail backpacker. 3rd ed. c2001.

ISBN 0-89732-583-4

1. Hiking–Appalachian Trail–Guidebooks. 2. Backpacking–Appalachian Trail–Guidebooks. 3. Appalachian Trail–Guidebooks. I. Logue, Frank, 1963– II. Logue, Victoria, 1961– Appalachian Trail backpacker. III. Title.

GV199.42.A68L64 2004

796.51'0974–dc22

2004059281

Cover design by Palace Press International, Inc.

Text design by Palace Press International, Inc. and Annie Long

Photos by Victoria and Frank Logue, Travis Bryant, and Russell Helms

Illustrations by Travis Bryant

Menasha Ridge Press

P.O. Box 43673

Birmingham, AL 35243

www.menasharidge.com

Appalachian Trail Conservancy

P.O. Box 807

Harpers Ferry, WV 25425

www.appalachiantrail.org

the

APPALACHIAN
trail HIKER

formerly
THE APPALACHIAN TRAIL BACKPACKER

Trail-proven advice for hikes of
any length

FOURTH EDITION

Victoria and Frank Logue

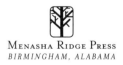

MENASHA RIDGE PRESS
BIRMINGHAM, ALABAMA

APPALACHIAN TRAIL CONSERVANCY
HARPERS FERRY, WEST VIRGINIA

ACKNOWLEDGMENTS

WE REMAIN THANKFUL TO THE MANY HIKERS WHO HAVE USED THEIR THOUSANDS OF MILES OF EXPERIENCE ON THE A.T. TO HELP SHAPE THIS BOOK THROUGH THE THREE PREVIOUS EDITIONS.

For this fourth edition, we would like to particularly thank Laurie Potteiger of the Appalachian Trail Conservancy for her ongoing assistance, both with this book and in the many others ways in which she educates and encourages A.T. hikers. We would also like to thank the following hikers who have completed the A.T. at least once in recent years who generously offered their feedback to this revised edition: Chris Bagby, Alan Beck, Steve Bekkala, Dennis and Mary Ann Giancola, and Lamar and Robert Powell. We are thankful for their assistance in keeping this book up to date so that it can be as helpful as possible to new generations of A.T. hikers. Any errors which remain are our own.

Contents

Chapter One

Following the Blazes

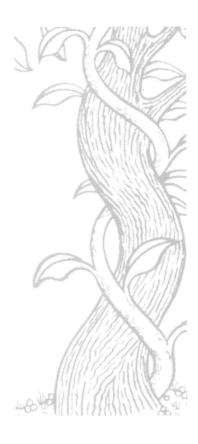

Following the blazes. There is a sense of mystique to that simple phrase that brings to mind the expedition of Lewis and Clark or the travels of William Bartram. Imagine wandering off into the woods to face the unknown, perhaps discovering things as yet undiscovered. At the very least, the Appalachian Trail (A.T.) offers you an introduction to nature in both her splendor and glory as well as her very worst.

A BRIEF HISTORY OF THE
APPALACHIAN TRAIL

The Trail, which winds through the Appalachian Mountains of 14 Eastern states, was the vision of Benton MacKaye (Kaye rhymes with sky) and others who had kicked around the idea for more than ten years. In 1921, MacKaye took the initiative and proposed the project in an article in *The Journal of the American Institute of Architects.*

MacKaye's original intent was to construct a pathway that would create an opportunity for American families to commune with nature. His trail would extend from "the highest peak in the North to the highest peak in the South, from Mount Washington (New Hampshire) to Mount Mitchell (North Carolina)." His plan had four parts: 1) to create the trail itself, 2) to build a series of shelters, 3) to create community camps, and 4) to build food and farm camps located along the trail's length. Although MacKaye's larger economic plan for the Appalachian Trail never gained support, it is nevertheless the reason for the Trail's existence today. With a continuous trail in easy reach of major cities, MacKaye argued,

> *"There would be a chance to catch a breath, to study the dynamic forces of nature and the possibilities of shifting to them the burdens now carried on the backs of men. . . Industry would come to be seen in its true perspective—as a means in life and not as an end in itself."*

Less than a year after MacKaye's article appeared in the architectural journal, the New York–New Jersey Trail Conference began work on a new trail with the goal of making if part of the A.T. In the Hudson River Valley, the newly built Bear Mountain Bridge would connect the future New England trail with Harriman State Park and, eventually, Delaware Water Gap in Pennsylvania.

Seeing that trail work had begun, in 1925 MacKaye and others formed the Appalachian Trail Conference to help guide the volunteers completing the Trail. During the next ten years, over 1,900 miles of partially connected trail were completed. In 1936 Myron H. Avery (who would lead the Appalachian Trail Conference for 20 years as president) finished measuring the flagged route of the Appalachian Trail and became the first 2,000-miler a year before the completion of the Trail.

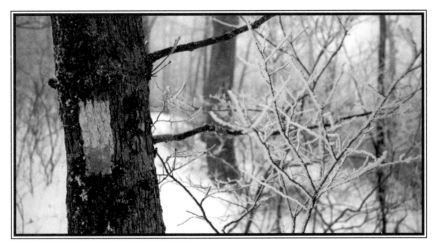

White Blaze of the Appalachian Trail

On August 14, 1937, Civilian Conservation Corps (CCC) workers cleared the final link in the 2,025-mile-long A.T. On a high ridge connecting Spaulding and Sugarloaf mountains in Maine, a six-man CCC crew cut the last two miles of trail. The route of the Trail was not as originally envisioned by MacKaye; it was longer—stretching from Mount Oglethorpe (the southern terminus of the Appalachians) in Georgia to Katahdin in Maine's Baxter State Park.

The A.T. met with misfortune the following year; a hurricane demolished miles of trail in the Northeast. Meanwhile, the decision to extend Skyline Drive in Virginia (under construction at the time) with yet another scenic route—the Blue Ridge Parkway—displaced 120 more miles of the recently completed route. It wouldn't be until the world settled down to rest from World War II that the trail would once again be made continuous.

In April of 1948, Earl Shaffer packed his Mountain Troop rucksack and headed for Georgia. "The Long Cruise," as Shaffer referred to his trip, started on Mount Oglethorpe and ended some 2,050 miles and four months later on top of Katahdin. Shaffer, who had fought in the Pacific during World War II, undertook the continuous "thru-hike" to "walk the war out of my system," as he would later write. His hike earned him the distinction of being the A.T.'s first thru-hiker.

In 1948, many considered Shaffer's thru-hike a stunt, but the dream of long-distance hiking spawned other long-distance trails, including the Pacific Crest Trail, which runs from Mexico to Canada, and the Continental Divide Trail, which follows the Continental Divide from Mexico to Canada.

Since 1948, when Shaffer's lone expedition carried him across construction- and hurricane-torn trail, the A.T. has seen many changes. Each year the Trail undergoes relocations and other improvements to its route, causing the trail's distance to change almost annually. From the original 2,025 miles it has stretched to more than 2,100 miles.

Legislation passed in 1968 and 1978 gave the National Park Service the power (and the money) to purchase and protect a corridor of land from Springer Mountain in Georgia to Katahdin's Baxter Peak. Less than one half of one percent of the trail remains unprotected.

Millions of people visit the Appalachian Trail annually. Whether spending a day hiking along its trails or half a year attempting to thru-hike its length, they are still inspired by MacKaye's dream of following the blazes.

A BRIEF TOUR OF THE APPALACHIAN TRAIL

The Appalachian Trail's southern terminus is on Springer Mountain in Georgia. With a total of 75.4 miles, Georgia's trail elevation ranges from 2,510 feet to 4,461 feet (Blood Mount Shelter). Georgia's brief section of trail is characterized by short, steep ups and downs. Although rising at times to elevations of over 4,000 feet, the Trail is mostly along undulating ridges at elevations of about 3,000 feet. The weather is comparable to lower elevations in northern Virginia and Maryland. Those tempted by the southerly latitude to plan spring break hikes in March may encounter sleet or snow. In federally designated wilderness areas (about half of the Trail in this state) authorities request hikers to camp out of sight of the Trail. The A.T. is crowded with thru-hikers in March and the first half of April.

The Trail crosses the state line into North Carolina at Bly Gap. The total trail mileage in North Carolina is 88.1 miles, plus an additional 154.9 miles passing along the Tennessee–North Carolina border. Once the A.T. crosses into North Carolina, it ascends steeply into the Nantahala National Forest with its mile-high peaks. From the Nantahala, the hiker heads north over the Stecoah Mountains to Great Smoky Mountains National Park. The A.T. reaches its highest elevation in the Smokies. At 6,643 feet, Clingmans Dome is the north-bounder's first taste of boreal forest with its balsam firs and rarely seen mountain cranberries. North of the Smokies, the A.T. crosses several bald mountains. These peaks are breezy realms of grass and sky where the hiker is rewarded by impressive 360-degree views. The Trail continues along the North Carolina–Tennessee border until it reaches Roan Mountain. The A.T. swings into Tennessee for good at a point roughly 25 miles north of Roan Mountain along a newly added route that contributes another waterfall to the scenery.

Only 137.9 miles of the Appalachian Trail pass through Tennessee (in addition to the 154.9 miles shared with the North Carolina border as mentioned above). From Grassy Ridge, the Trail descends into Laurel Fork Gorge, with its breathtaking waterfall, and crosses the dam at Watauga Lake before traversing a long ridge (known to thru-hikers as the Tennessee Turnpike) into Virginia.

The total trail mileage for Virginia is 549 miles (including 23.8 miles along the Virginia–West Virginia border). One quarter of the Appalachian Trail lies in Virginia, rang-

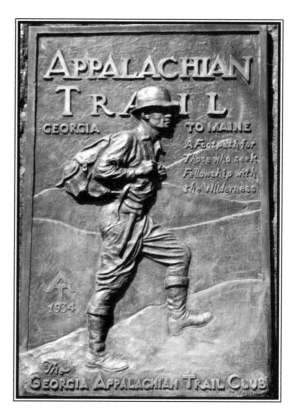

Springer Mountain plaque

ing in elevation from 668 feet to 5,500 feet. In addition to comprising a quarter of the Trail, this state encompasses such varied terrain and offers such different hiking experiences that we have divided it into four regions, corresponding to the four guidebooks published for this state by the Appalachian Trail Conservancy.

After leaving Tennessee, the A.T. enters the Southwest Virginia region, and shortly thereafter, the Trail town of Damascus, where the annual Trail Days festival celebrating the thru-hiking experience is held. The Trail passes through the open meadows of the Mount Rogers high country (5,000 feet and above) with a stunning seasonal display of rhododendron blooms.

Crossing over the New River and passing into the Central Virginia region, hikers travel over several noteworthy 3,000- to 4,000-foot peaks, including Dragon's Tooth, McAfee Knob, the Priest, Three Ridges, and Humpback Rocks.

Reaching Rockfish Gap, the A.T. enters the 107-mile Shenandoah National Park section. Gentle grades, climbs rarely exceeding 1,000 feet, an abundance of wildlife, and roadside amenities along nearby Skyline Drive are the highlights of this section. The Trail finally enters the Northern Virginia stretch comprised of low ridges, usually between 1,000 and 2,000 feet.

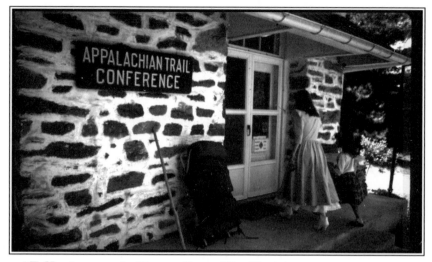

A.T. Headquarters in Harpers Ferry, West Virginia

The A.T. leaves the longest state to enter the shortest: West Virginia. With only 4 miles of trail, West Virginia still manages to pack in nearly 1,000 feet of elevation change from 265 feet at the Potomac River Footbridge to 1,200 feet at Loudoun Heights. The Trail passes through the historic town of Harpers Ferry, providing opportunities to explore the Harpers Ferry National Historical Park and its interpretive exhibits. As it leaves the town, heading south, the Trail follows a wooded ridge above the Shenandoah River, passing Jefferson Rock overlook, with impressive views of the Potomac and Shenandoah rivers. The Appalachian Trail Conservancy headquarters is located in Harpers Ferry, on a quarter-mile blue-blazed trail off the A.T.

After crossing the Potomac River, hikers enter Maryland and its 40.5 miles of trail. Maryland ranges in elevation from 230 feet at the C&O Canal Towpath to 1,880 feet at Quirauk Mountain.

The Trail through Maryland is gentle, with no climbs over 1,000 feet. Once you have climbed Weverton Cliffs, it may be the easiest state to hike (other than West Virginia). This section is a good place to find out if you're ready for more rugged parts of the Trail; for example, it's a great place to shakedown your body and gear without the tough climbs. The state requires hikers to stay at designated shelters and campsites while passing through Maryland.

The A.T. follows the crest of South Mountain Ridge into Pennsylvania with its 229.4 miles of trail. Here hikers will find the approximate halfway point of the Trail. Although the true midpoint changes from year to year, those attempting a thru-hike, or who have been hiking the A.T. in sections, usually celebrate here by consuming a half-gallon of ice cream at Pine Grove Furnace State Park.

The A.T. meets the end of the Blue Ridge Mountains in Pennsylvania at White Rocks, its northern terminus. It then descends into the Cumberland Valley.

The third largest of the A.T. states, Pennsylvania, is famous for its rocks. Trail maintenance clubs in this state joke about sharpening the rocks to torture hikers, and there are some areas (in particular, from Wind Gap to Fox Gap) that are reminiscent of walking on a bed of nails. After crossing the Susquehanna River at Duncannon, the Trail follows the eastern ridge of the Alleghenies to Delaware Water Gap.

From Delaware Water Gap, the A.T. enters New Jersey and its 72.4 miles of trail. The New Jersey section ranges from 350 feet at the Delaware River Bridge to 1,685 feet at High Point State Park viewpoint, near High Point Monument, which is the high point for the State of New Jersey. More wooded and removed from civilization than one might expect considering its proximity to large population centers, this section of the A.T. includes views of farmlands and pastures. Although the terrain is sometimes rocky, the elevation changes are generally moderate. A highlight of the southern section is glacial Sunfish Pond.

From the Kittatiny Mountain range, the Trail proceeds north through New York's 88.5 miles of trail. New York boasts the lowest point on the Appalachian Trail at 124 feet, located at the Trailside Museum and Zoo at Bear Mountain. The A.T. also climbs to a respectable 1,433 feet at Prospect Rock. New York's Trail, like the footpath in neighboring New Jersey, is more wooded and removed from civilization than visions of New York City might lead one to expect. The elevation changes are generally moderate, and vary from relatively flat and gentle to short, steep rocky pitches. Many rocky ledges provide valley and lake views.

Continuing northward, the Trail crosses back and forth, then enters Connecticut for good on top of Schaghticoke Mountain. Most of the 51.6 miles of trail are spent rambling along the Housatonic River and the Taconic Mountains. The trail ranges in elevation from 260 to 2,316 feet at Bear Mountain. This area of the A.T. is noted for accessible water, particularly in contrast to dry mid-Atlantic states of Maryland through New York. There are more walks along rivers than any other area. Several summits and ledges provide views, as opposed to the ridgewalking that characterizes the mid-Atlantic states. Ascents are not sustained; most are moderate, but with steep, fairly challenging sections that are short in duration and offer fine pastoral views.

In Sage's Ravine, the A.T. leaves Connecticut for Massachusetts and its 90.2 miles of the Trail. Having left the lower elevations of the mid-Atlantic states, the Trail continues to gain in elevation. From a low point of 650 feet at Massachusetts Route 2, it climbs to 3,491 feet at Mount Greylock. This area of the A.T. is also noted for its proximity to water, such as the Housatonic and Hoosic

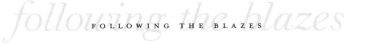

rivers, and scenic Upper Goose Pond. The Trail then passes through the Housatonic Valley, an area rich in American history. Several summits and ledges provide views of the bucolic countryside, particularly in the southern part of the state. The Trail is mostly moderate, but with steep, fairly challenging sections that are short in duration.

Just north of Williamstown, Massachusetts, and its famous summer theater, the A.T. enters Vermont. The Appalachian Trail and the Long Trail join at the Vermont border to follow the crest of the Green Mountains and its skiing areas for 104.1 miles. After descending Killington Peak at Sherburne Pass, the A.T. and the Long Trail climb together away from the road, then part ways. The A.T. continues another 45.6 miles along rugged woods and farmlands until it crosses the Connecticut River at Hanover, New Hampshire.

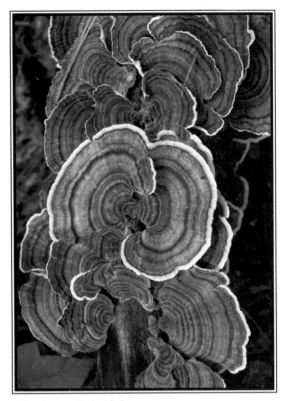

Turkey tail shelf fungus

After leaving Hanover, home of Dartmouth College, the Trail tops Smarts Mountain, then Mount Cube, and then Mount Mist. It ascends Mount Moosilauke, introducing the northbound hiker to the first above-tree-line climb on the Trail and the breathtaking White Mountains. Here, in the Presidential Range, the highest peak in the Northeast—Mount Washington—is a prize to conquer. At 6,288 feet, Mount Washington's hurricane-force winds and difficult-to-predict temperature drops earn the peak the odd boast of having the "worst weather in the world." The A.T. leaves New Hampshire, with its 161 miles of Trail, to enter Maine.

Maine holds the northern terminus for the Appalachian Trail at the end of its 281.4 miles. The A.T. in Maine is generally considered the most difficult of the 14 states, ranging in elevation from 490 feet at the Kennebec River to 5,267 feet at Katahdin.

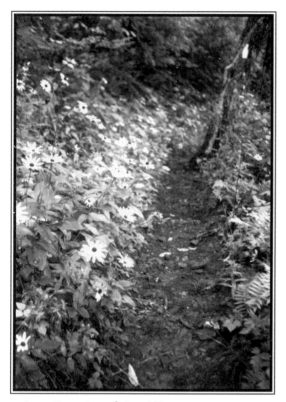
A small portion of the A.T.

Although the elevations seldom top 4,000 feet, the treadway is far rougher and steeper than all other areas of the Trail except for the White Mountains of New Hampshire. Some sections require grabbing onto tree roots and limbs to climb or descend, and are especially slippery and hazardous when wet. Switchbacks and graded trails are uncommon. In the Mahoosuc Range of western Maine and on some of the other rugged mountains, even the strongest hikers may average only 1 mile an hour. And while a small creek may be bridged elsewhere on the A.T., almost all streams and rivers in Maine must be forded. Highlights include crossing the Kennebec River on a free ferry and, of course, reaching Katahdin.

When hiking along the Appalachian Trail, you will generally find the following to be true of the terrain:

- The South has the highest mountains on the Trail, but those mountains have deep soils that allow for switchbacks. Lengthy, graded ascents and descents are frequent.

- The mid-Atlantic states have the lowest mountains, where the A.T. frequently leads along rocky ridges.

- In New England, the Trail is both rocky and steep, sometimes muddy and root-obstructed as well.

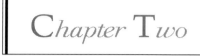

Chapter Two

The Trail Kitchen

One of the best things about hiking is that the food almost always tastes good. From a simple day hike with a picnic lunch to those greedily consumed calories during a long-distance trek, part of the outdoor experience always includes the meal. And why not? Food, water, and shelter are the basic necessities of life, and the exertion of a hike always adds a little spice to the meal. In this chapter, we'll look at the many food options available to the hiker, then turn to the kitchen itself—what types of stove and cooking tools are available, as well as good clean-up routines and a few other odds and ends.

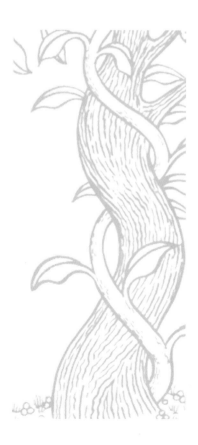

F O O D

From gallons of ice cream to All-You-Can-Eat (AYCE) buffets, long-distance hikers consume copious amounts of food whenever they hit a town near the Trail. And, because they can't take all that glorious food with them, they often leave dreaming about the Epicurean delights the next town might have to offer. For those on smaller-scale hikes and for ultralight backpackers, calorie intake is not as much of a concern. But, because packing light is important no matter the hiking distance, hikers must often accept a less-than-satisfying amount of food in tow.

D E H Y D R A T E D / F R E E Z E - D R I E D F O O D S

Like most hikers we usually stick to the low-cost supermarket brand dinners such as Kraft, Lipton, and a few others. Thanks, no doubt, to the number of families with working parents, supermarkets are filled with many easy-to-fix, just-add-water dinners. But specialty dehydrated foods designed for backpackers have come a long way too. Though still expensive, they offer variety to the macaroni-and-cheeses and ramen-noodle dinners many hikers subsist on.

We decided to test a few of the specialty dinners available on the market, and were pleasantly surprised by what came out of our cook pot. For breakfast, we tried an omelet with potatoes and sautéed onions. The two-serving egg dish was not a bad buy. A bit of a pain to clean up, but it definitely adds variety to the staples of oatmeal and toaster pastries.

For supper, we tried a dinner described as "turkey, vegetables, and wild rice in a tangy sour-cream sauce." The no-cook entrée (not actually true—when you hike, even boiling water is cooking) was actually quite tasty. The dinner says it serves two, although a hungry hiker would probably have to eat the entire dinner just to get halfway full. We also had freeze-dried ice cream for dessert. The two-serving portion of Neapolitan ice cream was good but expensive—and too small for a single hungry hiker. We were intrigued by the dried ice cream but we definitely recommend sticking to the cobblers, pies, and more filling desserts.

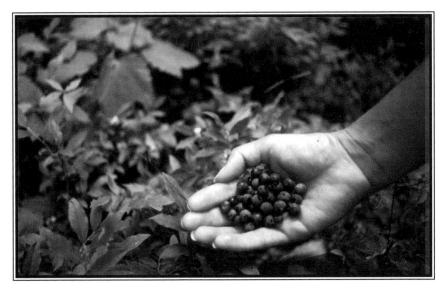

Wild blueberries on the A.T.

Among the companies that supply backpackers with dehydrated and freeze-dried foods are Adventure Foods, Alpine Aire, Harvest Foodworks, Mountain House, Natural High, Nature's Pantry, Richmoor, Trail Wise, and Wee Pack.

A new type of trail food, boxed in tiny "milk" cartons, is manufactured by Taste Adventure. These vegetarian, dehydrated meals are inexpensive and prepare quickly—just add boiling water and stir. We tried both the black-bean chili and lentil soup, which were tasty and provided large portions for two people.

Although we would still not recommend relying solely on these specially dehydrated and freeze-dried foods, we do believe they are a wonderful way to add variety to the diet. Keep in mind, though, that main dishes tend to cost two to three times as much as store-bought macaroni, pasta salads, and rice dishes. However, long-distance hikers can benefit from bulk purchasing online to get a much lower per-unit cost than is typically available in stores.

On the other hand, if you are willing to dehydrate food yourself, the sky's the limit. Although it takes time and effort, dehydrating your own food is a very inexpensive alternative. Dehydrators can be purchased through most outdoors stores and start at $50, though you can certainly use your own stove. All manner of food can be dehydrated—fruit, meats, and vegetables. *Trail Food* by Alan S. Kesselheim, published by Ragged Mountain Press, is a good resource for home dehydrators.

FRESH FOOD

With a little planning, weekend hikers can easily enjoy fresh foods. If you are willing to carry the weight of fresh meat and produce, again the sky is the limit. Steaks, hamburgers, fish, or chicken are all possible candidates to cook over your grill. And if you intend to have meat your second night out, freeze it before you go. By the end of the second day, it should be thawed and ready to cook. Make sure you keep it in a zipper-lock bag, or you could end up with a messy backpack. One of the greatest advantages of short hikes is that your diet is limited only by the amount of time you want to spend cooking.

Fresh foods are certainly an option for the long-distance hiker, although you can't rely solely on fresh foods for your backpacking diet—you have to eat these goodies your first night back on the trail after a shopping stop or face rotten and decaying food. We usually stick to hot dogs (turkey or chicken) on longer hikes, because they are the only meat that won't drip blood all over our packs; if you do buy chicken, steak, or some other meat, make sure it is wrapped well before you leave. Hot dogs roasted over a fire with some cheese make a delicious meal alternative, and you don't have to worry about ketchup, mustard, etc. We also occasionally carry apples, oranges, pears, carrots, and other fruits and vegetables that are not easily bruised.

LIVING OFF THE LAND

Unless you know your edible wild plants backward and forward, stick to store-bought and homemade foods when backpacking. Many edible plants can be easily confused with poisonous plants.

While attending a lecture on mushrooms, we were dismayed to find that a mushroom we had feasted on in Maine was potentially fatal. This mushroom has the color and taste of lobster and is parasitic, growing off both a safe and a very dangerous mushroom. Obviously, we had been lucky and decided we'll never take a chance like that again.

There are some obvious edibles, though. Blueberries grow profusely in the wild and are great in pancakes, on cereal, in oatmeal, and so on. Blackberries, gooseberries, currants, raspberries, and wild strawberries can also be found trailside. Mulberries, unless fully ripe, can be dangerous. Another safe wild plant is the ramp or wild leek. Its strong onion odor distinguishes it—use as you would an onion.

NUTRITION

W hether you carry fresh or dehydrated food, you want to make sure you have a well-balanced meal. However, getting proper nutrition on the trail is often a "Catch 22," particularly for the long-distance hiker. The more food you carry to meet your caloric needs, the heavier your pack. The heavier your pack, the more calories you burn. The more calories you burn, the more food you need to carry. It's a vicious cycle. While it is easy enough to carry sufficient food to account for calories burned during a day or weekend hike, it is difficult and often impossible to do so for extended trips.

Typical hikers burn close to 5,000 calories per eight-hour day on a back-packing trip, so it is important that the food you carry has high nutritional value for its weight. The three sources of nutrition include carbohydrates (simple and complex), fats, and proteins. Each of these sources address the short, medium, and long-term energy needs of the body.

Carbohydrates are either simple (table sugar, honey, molasses) or complex (cereals, bread, pasta, rice, fruit, and vegetables). The extra boost of energy you get after eating a candy bar comes from the simple carbs. However, if you relied solely on these, you would quickly lose energy and crash. When the simple carbs are used up, the body turns to the complex carbs for more sustained energy. This is why a lot of runners carbo-load before a big race, to ensure they have enough energy to finish. Carbohydrates, simple and complex, should make up about 50 to 60 percent of the backpacker's daily caloric intake.

When the body runs out of carbs, it turns to the fats stored in the body. This is why long-distance hikers lose weight—the amount of carb intake cannot keep up with the daily nutritional needs of burning 5,000-plus calories each day. (*Note:* This does not apply to ultralightweight backpackers.) Though we limit fats in our daily lives, on the trail fats should make up 20 to 25 percent of our diet. Sources of fats include butter, nuts, cheeses, and meats.

The third critical component to nutrition is protein. Though protein does-n't directly give energy to the body, it is an important source of aminoacids—the building blocks of the body. Many of the fat foods contain proteins, though incomplete ones, so eating beans (lima beans, lentils, etc.) help complete the protein and give the body what it needs. Other sources include oat and wheat cereals, vegetables, and powdered milk. Proteins should make up 15 to 20 percent of your daily diet.

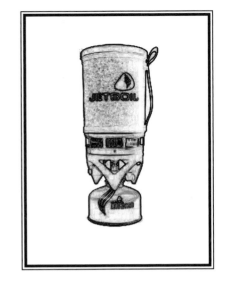

Jetboil

Getting the proper amount of carbohydrates, fats, and proteins is not all there is to good nutrition. You need to make sure you get the necessary minerals (calcium and iron among others) and vitamins. Food sources high in calcium are particularly important to long-distance hikers because of the amount of stress to your skeletal system, particularly your legs. Powdered milk and milk products such as cheese and sardines in oil are good sources of calcium. You may also want to consider the powdered energy drinks available through nutrition stores like GNC. Dried fruit, though not particularly high in calcium content, can add greatly to the total calcium and vitamin A intake when eaten on a regular basis. Whether or not you should take vitamins on an extended trip is a matter of preference, but we recommend taking some sort of vitamin supplement on an extended trip, particularly vitamins C and B. It is hard to maintain a balanced diet under strenuous conditions, so a multivitamin is your best bet during a long-distance hike.

We know of backpackers who subsist on the same thing for every meal, seven days a week. Experts recommend that you vary your backpacking diet as much as possible. While it may not bother you to eat cold cereal for breakfast, gorp for lunch, and macaroni and cheese every night for dinner, your body may soon tire of it. The most important aspect of a varied diet is the guarantee that you will be getting all the nutrients your body needs to function efficiently.

If you have certain dietary restrictions or are a vegetarian, you will need to be particularly diligent in maintaining a balanced diet. See the appendices for cookbook and food suggestions.

A Few Things to Consider

When shopping for backpacking trips, consider four things before making your food list: the weight of the food, ease of preparation, taste, and cost. Each of these categories are of varying importance to different people.

While on the trail, you may want to put together lavish meals, ensuring that you have an appetizing reward at the end of the day, but your pack (and your back) can only carry so much. Fresh food certainly tastes better than freeze-dried, but it tends to be bulkier, heavier, and to spoil more quickly.

Ease of preparation is another important factor. After a long day of hiking, it is unlikely that you will want to spend hours preparing your meal. Read package labeling before purchasing a food product. How long will it take to prepare? How long do you want to wait? On days when we reach our destination early, we usually don't mind waiting 20 minutes for our lentils and rice to simmer. Other days, we can hardly wait for the macaroni to finish cooking, and have eaten it a bit more al dente than we usually like. Buying food with various preparation times (an emphasis on the short side) will give you some options when you stumble into camp for the night.

Taste is something else to think about when purchasing food. If you can't stomach peanut butter at home, you probably won't like it in the outdoors, especially if you're forced to eat it. If you are unsure whether a certain backpacking food will be savory to you, try it before you hike. There is nothing worse than facing an unpalatable meal after a tough day's hike.

Finally, backpacking food (as with anything) can cost as much or as little as you like. From the expensive, extra-lightweight, specially packaged foods to the inexpensive homemade alternative, the backpacker has many choices. You know how much you have to spend. Once again, the key is diversity. Don't buy a week's worth of blueberry pancakes and lasagna; round it out with eggs and toaster pastries, macaroni and cheese, pasta salad, lentils, etc.

THE MENU

Hikers can get quite creative in putting good, simple, and quick meals together. We've listed below some of the foods we have enjoyed during our years of backpacking. With a few exceptions, most of them keep indefinitely. Add fresh vegetables or meat to the mix if the circumstances allow.

BREAKFAST

Breakfasts are easier to choose than lunches since there are so many breakfast products on the market. Most are vitamin-fortified, a gimmick to make mothers feel that they are providing a healthy breakfast for their child even when the product is stuffed-full of sugar. However, the extra carbohydrates, vitamins, and minerals are an added boon for hikers!

Cold cereal with powdered milk

Oatmeal (there are dozens of quick oatmeals now on the market)

Toaster pastries (such as Pop Tarts)

Eggs (will keep for several days)

Canned bacon

Bread with peanut butter

Bagels with cream cheese (cheese also keeps for several days)

Snickers or other candy bars

Granola bars

Gorp in powdered milk

Pancakes (bring the dry mix, add powdered milk and water)

Granola in powdered milk

Instant hash browns

Instant grits

Cream of Wheat

Bacon bars

English muffins

Breakfast bars (such as Nutrigrain Breakfast Bars)

Raisin bread

LUNCH

Lunches are always a problem for us, both at home and on the trail. Unless it is really cold, we never feel like taking the time to cook a lunch; but on the trail, there are only so many things you can do to improvise a cold lunch. We recommend that you do what suits you best. Some people hike better after a big, hot meal, but most do fine with a simple repast. How hot or cold it is may also determine your midday meal. When it is cold, we often choose to keep moving, eating snack foods while we hike, rather than stopping to prepare a meal.

Cheese

Nuts

Complex-protein bars

Cookies

Crackers (a number of varieties can be purchased spread with cheese or peanut butter)

Beef jerky

Peanut-butter-and-jelly sandwiches

Dried soups

Candy bars

Pepperoni

Graham or other type cracker and peanut butter

Sausage (hard types like salami, summer sausage, etc.)

Apples, oranges, and other fresh fruit

Lipton noodles and sauce

English muffins

Bagels

Crackers

Peanut butter

Foil-pouched meats, such as tuna

Corned beef or spam

Hard-boiled eggs

Dried fruit (including rolls, bars, etc.—raisins are a good choice)

Cheese sandwiches (pita and tortilla wraps are great hiking breads—stuff them with salami and cheese for a calorie-packed sandwich)

Granola bars

Snack foods (Little Debbie, Hostess, etc.)

Gorp (a mixture of dried fruit, nuts, M&Ms, sunflower seeds, etc.)

Vienna sausages

Fruit cake

SUPPER

Supper will probably be your most time-consuming meal of the day. It is time to relax, settle down for the night, and enjoy the great outdoors. You no longer have to worry about whether or not you'll reach your goal for the day. Your camp is set. Dinner is your only concern. Despite the fact that many backpackers eat macaroni and cheese night after night, there are many alternatives when choosing dinner on the trail.

Lentils

Instant rice dishes (instant gravies and cheese sauces can be added)

Macaroni and cheese (add canned or dry meat or dried soup)

Lipton noodle dinners

Instant mashed potatoes

Stove Top or other stuffings

Chef Boyardee spaghetti

Instant soup

Ramen noodles

Pasta salads

Couscous

SUPPER ALTERNATIVES

Pilafs (such as lentil, wheat, and rice)

Instant potato dinners (au gratin, etc.)

Tuna and other foil-pouched meats

Pepperoni, dried beef, sausages

Specialty dehydrated meals

SPICES AND CONDIMENTS

Not everyone uses spices, and no one carries all of those indicated below; but those who bring spices tend to use a variety. For their weight, spices and condiments can add a lot to a meal. Single serving packs are available in stores and in even more variety when you shop online.

Special containers to carry spices can be purchased through outdoor retailers and even at discount stores such as Wal-Mart. Don't use film containers, which contain harmful chemicals that might leach into your spices.

Garlic (dried or powdered)

Salt

Pepper

Italian seasoning

Seasoned butter

Tabasco

Red pepper

Curry powder

Chili powder

Oregano

Basil

Cumin

Onion powder

Squeeze margarine (lasts approximately one week in hot weather and almost indefinitely in cold weather)

BEVERAGES

Keeping hydrated is a very important part of hiking. Becoming dehydrated will seriously impair your body's ability to perform normal functions. The best thing to drink is water, but powdered drink mixes are a good way to add variety. The next-best thing to water is an electrolyte solution such as Gatorade or Gookinaid ERG. These help replace the electrolytes as well as the water that you lose while hiking. Some physiologists debate this claim and believe that electrolyte solutions do more harm than good. Other powder drinks, like Kool-Aid or Lipton Iced Tea mix, simply add variety.

There are very few of us willing to give up our morning cup of coffee when we hit the trail. If you do drink coffee or cocoa (unless decaffeinated), keep in mind that they are diuretics and you will need to drink more water to compensate.

Water

Powdered fruit drinks

Powdered iced tea

Powdered fruit teas

Jell-O mix (used as a tasty, hot drink that also supplies extra calories)

Instant coffee

Non-dairy creamer (for tea or coffee)

Powdered spiced cider

Powdered eggnog

Gatorade (powdered)

Gookinaid E.R.G.

Spiced cider

Hot tea

Cocoa/hot chocolate

ALCOHOL

There is something that is missing from the food list, and it's the one thing on which hikers tend to spend a lot of money—alcohol. We don't intend to preach—personally, there is nothing better to us than an ice-cold beer on a hot summer's day. Unfortunately, during the past decade or so hikers drinking alcoholic beverages have gotten out of hand a number of times. The result is that hikers are no longer allowed in certain places. Fortunately, most thru-hikers are very well thought of; but it is always the few who ruin things for all.

DESSERTS

Desserts are a nice way to finish your evening meal. They supply you with a few extra calories and help fill that last empty spot in your belly. They also make dinner special. Although pudding is a favorite, there are a number of easy-to-make desserts on the market.

Instant puddings

Instant cheesecakes

Cookies

Instant mousse

Jell-O or other flavored gelatins

Powdered milk (mostly used to add to other foods)

Snack cakes

Easy-bake cakes

Specialty dehydrated desserts

TRAIL SNACKS

We're not snackers at home, but we find snacking important when hiking. Because you don't want to stuff yourself at meals—for comfort's sake as well as due to the fact that a too-full stomach can make you drowsy—it is a good idea to snack on high-energy food during breaks and while hiking. One of the most popular trail snacks is gorp, a mixture of nuts, dried fruit, and M&Ms. Actually, gorp can consist of anything you like, but the following is a list of some popular ingredients. Mix and match your favorites: peanuts, almonds, pecans, walnuts, filberts, cashews, M&Ms, Reese's pieces, shredded coconut, chopped dates, raisins, banana chips, dried pineapple, figs, prunes, sunflower seeds, and cereals like Cheerios.

Other trail snacks include: hard candy, Skittles, semisweet chocolate, mixed nuts, fruit bars and rolls. There are many packaged snack bars on the market these days. Use your imagination. As long as it is within easy reach and will keep in the outdoors for more than a day, it will make a good snack. Remember too that "snacks" can round out dinners and often make up your entire lunch.

FOOD FOR EXTENDED HIKES

If you are hiking for more than a week, it's doubtful that you will be able to or want to carry enough food to last you. You will need to find another way to supply your nutritional needs. There are two basic solutions: buy your food along the way or send provisions ahead. Much of this depends on where you are hiking along the Trail. These days hikers tend to purchase their food as they hike. The number of stores and hostels carrying food has increased in recent years, and food is particularly available during the months when northbounders (those hiking from Georgia to Maine) are on the Trail—usually spring through summer.

Check the *A.T. Companion*, a guide published annually by the Appalachian Long-Distance Hikers Association and the ATC, for updates on resupply options. Since 2000, a handful of supermarkets with wide selections have sprung up close to the A.T. On the other hand, smaller stores sometimes have high turnover and may go out of business. In general, resupply points are more frequent in the mid-Atlantic, less frequent in the far-northern and far-southern states. On average, hikers resupply every three to seven days.

The option to purchase food along the way eliminates the need to time your arrival in town to coincide with the hours of a post office. (It's nice not to have to depend on the U.S. Postal Service for food.) It also allows you to satisfy any sudden food cravings you may have! But for those who wish to send food ahead, a number of hostels and businesses in addition to post offices accept mail drops for hikers. A hiker can retrieve a package any day of the week and the establishment is usually open longer than the post office. Businesses, as opposed to the Postal Service, can accept packages shipped via UPS or other commercial carrier.

One more option involves shipping food ahead to yourself on the Trail. When you find yourself in a grocery store with a great selection and you know that paltrier choices lay ahead, you can buy some extra food to ship a bit farther up the Trail. Shipping costs are lower for the short Parcel Post trip, and the food should be waiting on you within three days. This offers a way to get around the problem of planning well in advance without having to depend on using only what is available trailside at the time you need it.

Burying caches of food is not an acceptable way to resupply yourself with food, as it is ecologically unsound.

Cooking Hygiene

Most gastrointestinal ailments do not come from waterborne problems. The more prevalent cause of sickness stems from not washing hands after going to the rest room and then handling food. An alcohol hand gel, such as Purel, used after going to the bathroom will eliminate this problem.

PACKING YOUR FOOD

PACKAGING AND REPACKAGING

Proper packing is essential and is only a problem if you are unable to repackage the food yourself. Don't buy rigid, heavyweight containers if they must go straight into your pack.

In the interest of space, weight, and waterproofing, you will want to repackage your food into plastic bags or some other sturdy, waterproof container. Hikers joke that the "yellow-and-blue-makes-green" Glad Lock zipper bags are one of the great backpacking inventions of our time. This might be a little exaggerated, but not much. Other options include reusable plastic, squeezable food tubes. A clip at the bottom is used to squeeze the food upward toward the spout. I have seen these used only for peanut butter and jelly; however, both peanut butter and jelly now come in plastic containers, so it is just as easy to use them in their containers.

Rigid plastic egg cartons are also available for less than $3 from most outdoors stores. They come in both the dozen and half-dozen size and are a wonderful way to carry eggs. These containers will hold small and medium-size eggs only. Unless you have room for food at the top of your pack where it won't get smashed, make sure the packaging is sturdy enough to survive the weight to which you intend to subject it.

To pack food for backpacking, sort your boxes and other packages into meals. Open the boxes and pour the contents into plastic bags of appropriate sizes. You do not need to do this with meals that come in foil or other waterproof pouches. On short trips, you can cut down on weight and space by adding the powdered milk, salt, pepper, etc. to the bag at home. If you need the directions, cut out the portion of the box where the recipe is written and put it in the bag with the meal.

Some food products do better in plastic bags with twist ties. If you are carrying powdered milk, for example, it is best to double bag it and shut it with a twist tie because the grains of milk tend to get caught in the zipper and keep it from closing properly.

Vacuum Sealing

Use of a vacuum sealer for packaging meals is becoming increasingly common. A typical sealer costs $50–$200 and can make repackaging of items at home a snap. A vacuum seal certainly beats a zip-locked bag when mailing foods ahead. Single-size meals or food items can be packed at home and shipped ahead. This is especially useful for hikers preparing their own dehydrated foods. Vacuum sealing is not limited to food items, however—you may use this method for some strongly scented items, including soaps and shampoos.

TRAIL KITCHEN EQUIPMENT

Unless you plan on taking bagels right out of the package and dipping them into cream cheese or lathering them with peanut butter, you probably want to cook your food. Though going stoveless is quick and convenient, nothing beats a hot meal, especially when the weather is cold.

Stoves

Backpacking doesn't have to be synonymous with macaroni and cheese or whatever you can throw into boiling water. With the advances in stove technology allowing you to simmer or bake food, your diet is limited only by your imagination and willingness to cook.

It's true that using a camp stove while backpacking is necessary in part due to the fact that in many areas fires are prohibited. Gone are the days of gobs of dough roasted on a stick over a blazing campfire. In areas where fires are permitted, the woods around shelters and campsites have often been picked clean of downed wood by other hikers. Foraging for firewood also damages plant life and removes an important part of the forest ecosystem, because the downed wood provides both food and shelter for forest insects and animals. For all these reasons, leave-no-trace guidelines recommend against campfires when possible. Fortunately, stoves are now lightweight and efficient as well as inexpensive. Regardless of what stove you take, test it at home before relying on it for a hike.

Backpacking stoves tend to be categorized depending on the type of fuel they burn. Broadly speaking, the two most common types of stoves used on the Trail today are white-gas and alcohol stoves. While stoves using other fuel sources, including kerosene and canister, remain in use, their fuel is not commonly found along the Trail and most A.T. hikers avoid them for longer hikes. One stove type worthy of a footnote burns fuel tablets such as the Esbit brand. While the fuel is not always readily available, these tabs can be shipped to you on the Trail, and overall fuel costs can be lowered by buying the fuel tabs in bulk.

WHITE-GAS STOVES

This has long been the liquid fuel of choice. Usually found under the name of "Coleman," the fuel comes in quart- or gallon-sized cans and can be found just about anywhere in North America. The flame it produces is hot, reliable, and relatively clean in almost all weather conditions, but only if you keep your stove properly primed and the fuel tank well pressurized. White gas evaporates quickly and the spilled fuel is very flammable. Stoves using white gas must be insulated from snow or frozen ground because the heat of the stove could thaw the ground and make your stove unstable.

White-gas stoves offer a number of features that you may want to consider before making a purchase. Depending upon the type of backpacking trips you intend to make, one option is to purchase a stove with a double burner. This allows you to cook two items simultaneously. The major drawback with the two-burner is that it adds a significant amount of weight to your pack. If you are traveling in larger groups, this could be a viable option, as equipment can be spread evenly throughout the group.

Push-button ignition or "piezo-ignition" is another stove feature, which means you can light your stove with the push of a button. Keep in mind, though, that the piezo can short out in the rain and that too much heat can actually melt the button. As long as you have a back-up plan—matches or a lighter—you won't have to worry too much if that happens.

Some stoves come with a repair kit, and for others you must purchase it separately. Either way, it is always a good idea to carry along a repair kit no matter how trustworthy you feel your stove is.

Most stoves come with a windscreen, either a stand-alone, wrap-around aluminum barrier that keeps the wind from whipping the flames on your stove or a small, half-inch band of metal that circles the stove's burner. The latter is less effective in high winds.

Fuel Bottles

A 16- to 22-ounce container of white gas generally lasts 7 to 12 days. In cold weather, because fuel consumption is slightly higher, you can count on no more than a week's worth of fuel from any 22-ounce container. In warmer weather, one container may last as long as two weeks.

There are a number of manufacturers of fuel bottles, but the most commonly used bottles are the MSR, Sigg, and Nalgene. The MSR fuel bottles can be purchased in three sizes: 11-ounce, 22-ounce, and 33-ounce, though the latter are probably not necessary for most hikes. Sigg offers a liter-size fuel bottle as well as sizes ranging from 8 ounces to 48 ounces. Both brands are made of noncorrosive aluminum and are relatively inexpensive. Fuel faucets are available for both the MSR and Sigg bottles. The screw-on cap allows you to turn the top to pour and turn again to seal without a leak. Nalgene bottles, which do not fit the MSR stoves, can also be purchased—pint size and quart size.

Operating and Maintaining Your Stove

- Carry a repair kit from your manufacturer and know how to use it. Practice taking your stove apart before you hike.
- Use a heat deflector and a windscreen to reduce fuel consumption. The windscreen also helps keep your flame steady. If you don't have a windscreen, use a piece of doubled aluminum foil.
- If you can't prime your stove directly, carry an eyedropper. You can extract the fuel from your fuel bottle with the dropper—much safer than pouring fuel from the bottle into the priming well.
- Don't fill white-gas stoves more than three-fourths full. The extra air space will help generate pressure.
- After each trip, empty the fuel from your stove. What you can't pour out, burn. Fuel left in stoves leaves residues that will clog your fuel jets and filters.
- Burning a cap of Gumout Carburetor Cleaner along with a half tank or half-a-pint of gas will help dissolve residues. Do this once a year to keep your stove clean.
- Residues also build up in your fuel source (Coleman fuel can) if you don't use it within a year. If your fuel is getting old, dispose of it. Don't put it in your stove. Call your local dump or landfill and ask them how to dispose of old fuel.
- You can hold on to your Coleman fuel longer if you store it in individual fuel bottles rather than the original gallon container. The fuel will stay cleaner longer and burn hotter and leave less soot on your pots. Keep your stove in a dust-free environment (such as a fabric sack) when it is not in use.

- By pre-filtering any low-grade fuel you might be using, you can avoid clogs and repairs later. Most manufacturers offer filters for their stoves, and Coleman sells an all-purpose, 1.5-ounce aluminum filtering funnel. This will filter fuel before it is stored in your fuel bottle. To conserve fuel, keep a lid on your pot whenever possible.

- When cooking on snow, make sure there is some sort of insulation beneath your stove so it doesn't sink.

ALCOHOL STOVES

More than 40 percent of long-distance hikers on the A.T. use alcohol stoves. Nearly impossible to find along the Trail prior to 1999, denatured alcohol is now ubiquitous. Alcohol, which is made from plant cellulose rather than petroleum, burns cleanly and is a nonvolatile fuel. Alcohol stoves have no moving parts, which eliminates the maintenance issues associated with white-gas stoves. Stove operation is much quieter, if less hot, than with white-gas stoves.

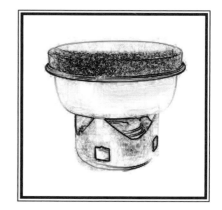

Trangia alcohol stove

Cook times are similar to those of gas stoves—an alcohol stove can bring two cups of cold water to boil in just five-and-a-half minutes. However, burn times are shorter (about nine minutes with two tablespoons of fuel), and hikers who opt for ultralightweight alcohol stoves stick with simpler boil-water-and-eat meals. Simmering is also an issue, being more difficult to control.

Using an Alcohol Stove

Alcohol stoves must be placed on a sturdy, noncombustible surface. Fill the stove with denatured alcohol to the desired level (often just a couple of tablespoons will do). Like other stoves, alcohol stoves function more effectively when used with a windscreen, and with lower burning temperatures this is even more important with them. The stove is lit by holding a match near the top center of the stove.

Alcohol stoves take about a minute to reach full cooking temperature. It may not look like the stove is lit until a pot is placed on it, but do not set the pot until you have allowed the stove to reach its full force. Do not attempt to put out the stove. Let the stove burn out the fuel on its own.

Allow the stove to cool completely before refueling. If you cannot hold the stove comfortably in your hands for at least ten seconds, it is still too hot to refuel. Only refuel from a small measuring cup to avoid exposing the full fuel bottle to a source of ignition.

Some hikers use methanol, found in hardware store paint departments as paint thinner. At gas stations and other stores methanol is sometimes sold with the brand name HEET as a gas-line antifreeze. The vaporization pressures are higher than those of ethanol so you should make sure that using this fuel source is recommended by your stove manufacturer before trying it out. Methanol is also very poisonous and should be handled with caution.

Do not use isopropyl alcohol as a fuel source. Though readily available as rubbing alcohol, isopropyl alcohol contains about 30 percent water. Though flammable, it burns less hotly than denatured alcohol and will blacken your pots with smoke.

Making Your Own Stove

While a variety of well-built, lightweight alcohol stoves are available through outdoor retailers, many hikers have opted to make their own "soda-can stove." Directions widely available online show how to turn aluminum cans (Pepsi and Budweiser brands work best) into an ultralightweight backpacking stove. Some basic tools and a bit of patience are all that is required to create your own alcohol stove. For less handy hikers, these stoves are also available for purchase.

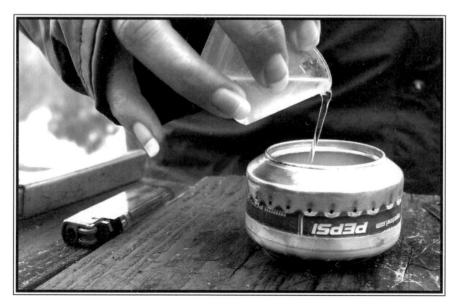

The Logues' homemade-style alcohol stove

Stove Safety

🍁 It's not a good idea to cook inside your tent or in any other unventilated space. Tents melt very easily, but even more dangerous is the fact that stoves use up oxygen and produce carbon monoxide, a sure way to a quick death. If you must cook in your tent, make sure it is well ventilated, or try cooking under the vestibule to avoid becoming ill (if not worse) from the fumes generated by the stove.

🍁 Since most stoves get very hot once lit, never set the stove directly on the floor of your tent. Instead, place it on a nonburnable pad such as a ceramic tile or a flat rock. Also, to avoid a tip-over, make sure your stove is firmly set before lighting . Do not move any type of stove while lit.

🍁 Never light a liquid-burning stove inside your tent. Flare-ups are very common and tent/sleeping bag materials are susceptible to flames as are your hair, eyebrows, beard, etc.

🍁 For alcohol stoves use only denatured alcohol.

🍁 Allow alcohol stoves to fully cool before refueling.

Accessories

Rather than relying on the heavier white-gas-style fuel bottles, alcohol may be carried in Nalgene containers. Sixteen ounces of alcohol will typically provide enough fuel for one hiker for five days on the Trail.

A pot cozy made of Styrofoam or other insulated materials can be fitted over the lidded cook pot after it has been removed from the stove. This keeps the food hot and allows the cooking to continue, while saving fuel. It also avoids risking burning food at the bottom of the pot.

BAKING ON THE TRAIL

It used to be that if you wanted to bake something while backpacking, you were going to have to carry along several pounds of stove. Traveling Light has made baking while backpacking an actual option with its Outback Oven. With the Ultralight, which uses your own cookpot for baking, you need only add seven ounces to your pack weight.

The Outback Oven uses the circulation of hot air in a convection dome to concentrate heat around the baking pan. Hot air vents out a hole in the top and a thermometer can be viewed through the hole to monitor the baking temperature. A riser bar separates the pan from the heat to prevent scorching and a stainless steel diffuser plate disperses heat from the stove. Finally, a reflector collar directs heat upward to boost the stove's efficiency.

Does it work? Yes, actually. We've used it with great success, adding a gourmet touch to our hikes. Should you take it on a backpacking trip? Sure, if the trip is short. However, on an extended trip, it's be too much trouble to lug and the ingredients to cook with just a tad too expensive.

ON GOING STOVELESS

Another not-quite-so-popular option is to eat only cold foods. I've met only a few hikers that depend on cold meals during their backpacking trips. It is not an impossible option, although most hikers can't live without their morning coffee, which, along with other hot beverages, is vital in cold, wet weather. Hikers who opt to go stoveless subsist for the most part on sandwiches—both cheese and peanut butter—along with toaster pastries, tuna, and cereal.

COOKWARE AND UTENSILS

The cooking pot may seem innocent, but it is one of the hiker's most important tools. It is a multiuse vessel used to boil water for drinks and meals, to gather water from a nearby source, to use as a bowl, and to hold your stove while hiking.

There are several options when it comes to choosing which material your cookware is made of:

ALUMINUM: Lightweight and generally inexpensive, aluminum is more prone to denting and scorching than steel. If you want to purchase aluminum, buy pots with a nonstick coating.

STAINLESS STEEL: These are more durable than aluminum but also heavier. Because of their slick surface, it is easier to keep them clean.

TITANIUM: This amazingly lightweight and strong metal may cut ounces but it is also expensive and prone to scorching.

COMPOSITE: These pots are usually made of fused aluminum and stainless steel, with the stainless steel on the inside to minimize sticking. While they offer a nice balance of weight and durability, they are more expensive than plain aluminum or stainless steel.

Among the features you might find when searching for the perfect cookset are the bail handle or swing handle, the black exterior finish, nonstick finish, a lipped rim, and rounded bottom edge.

The bail handle works fine on large pots but be careful if it falls against the side of the pot because the handle will conduct heat pretty quickly and unless you have a pot holder, you could be in for a nasty burn. Oddly enough, the swing handles, designed to eliminate that very problem, can get hot too. They swing out from the sides of the pot, but even the rubber-coated handles get pretty warm. Swing handles also make it hard to use a windscreen or to nest your pots. Your best bet: don't buy pots with handles at all. Instead, buy a handleless pot and use a pot grabber. If your set does not come with one, an inexpensive pot grabber can be purchased separately. Pot grabbers will keep you from burning your fingers and spilling your meal.

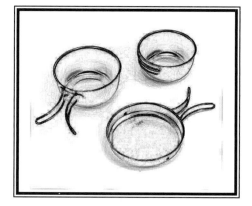

Cooking set
(Snow Peak Titanium Mini Solo)

Pots that have been given a black exterior finish tend to absorb heat faster and decrease the boiling time in your pot. Another option is to spray a pot you already own with flat black paint. You will achieve the same effect. As with your home cookware, camping pots with a nonstick finish make cooking and cleaning much easier. A nonstick finish is a must if you intend to bake.

A lipped rim is essential if you intend to use a pot grabber. Not only does it give the pot grabber something to hold onto, but it makes your pot stronger and less prone to warping. Pots with rounded bottom edges encourage the even distribution of heat up the sides of the pot and make cleaning a bit easier with no goopy corners to clean.

Although hikers use varying sizes of pots, you should choose your pot depending on your menu and the number of people in your group. The main thing is that you want to carry pots that are neither too small nor too big. I've met many hikers who found that one-liter pots tend to overflow during cooking, making cleanup a real chore. Improperly cleaned pots can lead to an uncomfortable hike: they increase your chance of food poisoning and serve as an irresistible lure to hungry animal neighbors in the night.

Still, if you hike solo and eat small meals, the smallest, one-liter, pot is probably fine for you, although only the smallest of stoves will nest in the pot.

Probably the ideal size for solo hikers and the smallest pot feasible for couples is the one-and-a-half-liter pot. Most stoves will nest in this pot, and it can accommodate enough pasta for two (or one really hungry hiker!).

Most couples we know carry nesting pots, the one-and-a-half- and two-liter pots nestle perfectly, and you can carry your stove in the one-and-a-half-liter pot. If your stove doesn't fit in the two-liter pot, it is too big. For our family of three, we use one pot to cook our dinner in and the other to mix drink (or to warm the drink when it's cold outside). A three-liter pot is really only necessary if you are cooking for a group of four or more. Many stove manufacturers offer special cooking pots to go with stoves.

COOKWARE TIPS

Before you head out into the woods with your new pots (or old ones), you might want to make some modifications to make cooking in the backcountry easier. If you have pots without a nonstick finish, try notching the inside walls of your pot at commonly used intervals such as one cup, two cups, three cups, and so on. This will help you measure the correct amount of water for rice or other meals that can be ruined by approximation. If you have a nonstick finish on your cookware, try painting a line on the outside of your pot.

If you use a frying pan and it doesn't double as a lid, you may want to solder a heat diffuser to the bottom of the pan. This will spread the heat more evenly across the bottom of the pan. Heat diffusers can be bought at most outdoor retailers.

UTENSILS

When it comes to carrying implements, hikers opinions are split. I usually carry a spoon, a bowl, and a pocketknife. A three-inch lock-blade pocket knife or a Swiss Army knife will prove adequate for most hikes, though hikers usually say they don't use these knives often. Some hikers prefer a fork, a spoon, and a pocketknife, and they use their cooking pot as a bowl. A spork (fork/spoon combination) is another option worth considering. Couples usually carry bowls, and few carry plates.

Cups are a matter of preference. We previously carried the Sierra-style cup that features indentations showing measurements, but we didn't really like them. Now we have switched to the increasingly popular thermal travel mug.

Extras, such as grills and coffee pots, are rarely used on longer hikes but may be worth their weight and bulkiness on short trips—if you drink a lot of coffee or intend to grill the fish you catch or the steaks you brought. And the coffee press is rapidly replacing the old-style percolator. For extended trips, most hikers stick to instant coffee and eat their steaks when in town to resupply.

CLEANING UP AFTER MEALS

C leaning pots, dishes, and utensils is an absolute necessity. Many hikers have found out the hard way that giving cleaning the short shrift can result in severe gastrointestinal problems. Dirty pots also beg for the appearance of pests such as raccoons, skunks, mice, and even bears (not to mention the hardships caused by dried-on macaroni and cheese, which is worse than super glue to clean up).

While in town, it might be good etiquette to leave a bit of food on your plate, but on the Trail it is always best to eat all your cooked food. Scraping out the last morsels from the dish will leave less to clean up. You could burn or bury the rest, but animals will be attracted to the scent. It's best for you and the animals with which you share the Trail to not scatter the scraps. If you do have left overs, you should pack them out with your trash to avoid trouble.

The best solution is to carry a little biodegradable soap and a pot scrubber. Here's one time-tested clean-up method. For hot meals, use two pots—the smaller pot to cook the food in and the larger to heat water and rinse dishes. After heating the water in the big pot, add the water to the entrée in the smaller pot. After you've eaten, add more water and some soap to the smaller pot to use as a wash-pan. The remainder of the hot water in the large pot becomes your rinse water. Use a little biodegradable soap (although soap isn't even necessary if you wash your pot with hot water and boil your next meal) and a pot scrubber.

Be sure to wipe pots and utensils clean and dry them out. Bacteria are not able to live on a dry surface for long. In fact, putting pots in the sun for an hour disinfects them, though that is an impractical clean-up routine. Boiling water for your next freeze-dried meal will sterilize anything that's left in the cooking pot.

Cleaning should be done 200 feet away from the campsite or shelter and far from the water source. Also remember to pack everything out.

CLEAN-UP TIPS

- Use a lid when boiling your water. Boiling time will be much faster and you will conserve fuel.

- Always strain out large food scraps and carry them out with you (to the next nearest trash receptacle).

- Never wash dishes within 200 feet of your water source, biodegradable soap or not. Dispose of your dishwater away from camp by spreading it over a large area rather than dumping it in one spot.

- Fill your biggest pot with water, heat it, and wash away. Warm, soapy water on a chilly night makes dish duty a bit more bearable.

- If you are part of a group of three-to-five hikers, try using a collapsible bucket. Fill it with clean rinse water for the final dip.

- If you lose your scrubbing sponge, substitute with your hiking partner's toothbrush. Just kidding. Try using ashes or sand, instead. They work great as an abrasive. Toss them in your pot and use your hand or a cloth to scrub them against the metal.

- If you absolutely cannot abide to the idea of doing dishes, confess your abhorrence but make sure you make up for it by taking on another chore.

- Short trip? Leave the soap behind and clean everything when you get home.

Use your sleeping bag as a cooler on hot days by inserting already cooled soft drinks or water into the middle or your bag. The liquid will stay cold for several hours.

Chapter Three

Water

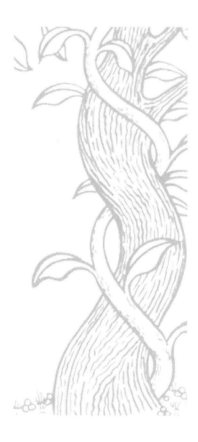

Water is essential for life. This simple fact seems innocuous when you are at home with an ample water supply. However, once you hit the Trail, much thought and planning needs to go into how and where you will find water that is safe to drink. Never deprive yourself of water—this leads to dehydration, which contributes to numerous ailments, including heat exhaustion, heat stroke, and hypothermia. Proper planning is the preventive for water woes. Where will you get water? How will you treat the water you do get? You must be able to answer these two questions before you hit the Trail, and the answers are just as important for the day hiker as they are for weekend backpackers and thru-hikers.

WHERE TO FIND WATER

The best source of information on water sources along the Appalachian Trail is the regional trail guides published by the Appalachian Trail Conservancy and some of the A.T. maintaining clubs. Another good, though less detailed, source of information is the ATC's annually updated *Data Book*. It is, of course, true that trail conditions change much faster than books, so you cannot always solely depend on the *Data Book* or guidebooks alone. Springs can run dry and are often intermittent. The same goes for small streams. Local trail clubs often post signs at shelters to let hikers know where the nearest water supply can be found. If there is not a sign, keep an eye out for a blue-blazed trail, particularly near a shelter. The blue blaze is often used to guide you toward a water source.

On the A.T. you will get your water from a variety of sources, including pumps, springs, and maybe even a beaver pond (yes, you actually get water from ponds and streams). One shelter even boasts a cistern. Water sources vary from stagnant pools dribbling from their source nearly half a mile away from the Trail (and downhill to boot!) to clear, ice-cold springs gushing in front of a shelter.

The higher you are the harder it will be to find water, although there are notable exceptions such as Lakes of the Clouds, in the Whites of New Hampshire, and Thoreau Spring, only a mile away from Katahdin's Baxter Peak. Conversely, the lower you are the more water there is, and the more likely it is that you will have to treat that water. Once again, there are exceptions to the rule. The awe-inspiring Potaywadjo Spring in Maine's lake country is one: the eight-foot round spring looks like a swimming pool compared to the paltry springs of the mid-Atlantic.

But on a hot day, even a beaver pond can look good, and it takes a lot of restraint not to dip your cup into the inviting liquid. Don't succumb to the urge to drink risky water before you've purified it. It is easier to carry an extra pound or two of water than suffer the discomforts of *Giardia* and other ailments that dehydrate you and cause you to lose your strength. Diarrhea and cramps are unpleasant at home and doubly so while hiking.

Collecting Water

Where you get your water will matter as much as how you treat it. Springs are almost always (but not always) a good choice for clean water; definitely better than a big river that's caught who knows what on its trip to the sea. Look around the spring first, though, as we have found rotting animal corpses near springs. With any water source, if there is anything even remotely animal-like nearby—beaver dam, animal scat—walk well upstream and look for an area clear of problems.

Much of water itself is clean. The problem, according to researcher Ryan Jordan of Montana State University's Center for Biofilm Engineering, is sediment at the bottom of streams and ponds, as well as the thin surface film on standing water, that contain the usual suspects listed below. The microbes grow in the slime to which scientists refer as biofilm. Let the surface film slip into your water bottle or stir up the sediment while filling your bottle, and you will gather biofilm clumps with your water. Jordan says that these biofilm clumps create a greater chance of sickness than drinking the same number of free-floating individual bacteria cells. The larger, attached groups of bacteria found in biofilm are more resistant to the helpful bacteria in your body that are the body's usual defense against these baddies. Biofilms are often no match for iodine tablets and can clog water filters.

Jordan's "best practices" for collecting water are to find a spot where you will not disturb the sediment, submerge a closed water bottle, open it under the surface, and let water flow in from the middle of the water source. Close the bottle while it is still submerged and lift it out. This technique will give you biofilm-free water. Even with this improved water-gathering technique, water treatment is required for all water on the Trail. Jordan's research highlights this fact. About five years ago, Jordan interviewed 120 hikers who had been on the A.T. for three months or more. Of the hikers he interviewed, 90 percent had suffered some gastrointestinal problems. Hikers out for shorter lengths of time are also not immune—Jordan found that 20 percent of the hikers had experienced those problems within the first week of their hike. His study also highlighted the extreme importance of washing your hands, especially after a trip to the bathroom.

How Much Should You Carry?

Like everything else, how much water you carry is up to you. One to two quarts per person is pretty standard when it comes to the amount of water carried constantly by hikers. Between the two of us, we carry two to three quarts most of the time, which is usually adequate. We can think of only a handful of times we were forced to eat cold meals for supper or go drinkless. Granted, there have been a few times we spent more than half an hour waiting to fill our canteens as water dripped from an improvised funnel, but that type of situation is rare.

WATER CONTAINERS

There are two basic choices when it comes to carrying water—whether to strap on a hydration system or stick to the time-tested water bottle.

The backpack hydration system consists of a collapsible water bladder that either comes as part of your pack (Kelty, Jansport, Mountainsmith, and others offer packs with hydration systems built in—usually a sleeve on the outside of a pack) or fits inside your pack. These include a flexible tube that you suck on to draw out the fluid. The bladders can hold up to two or three quarts.

Nalgene water bottles remain popular containers with their easy-to-fill wide-mouth design. They are available in a variety of sizes. The screw-on tops are also recommended. Some hikers wear special holsters that hold their bottles in an easy-to-reach position: no more stopping to get a drink! Also popular is the sports-type bottle with its screw-off cap and pull-out drinking spout.

A little more flimsy but still popular and viable alternative are empty plastic soda bottles. The one-liter size is used the most. They tend to leak a bit around the cap, but are great when a heat wave hits and you need to carry extra water for a limited time. They are also a low-cost lightweight option.

Something extra (but worth it) to carry is a collapsible water bag. This is a larger version of the Platypus-style water container. They're wonderful at camp because they hold more than enough water for dinner, cleanup, and sometimes even a sponge bath. Water bags, however, are unwieldy to carry filled in your pack as your only water holder.

Most distributors of water bags also sell shower attachments that connect to the spout. We've owned one but found ourselves never using it, as it always was either too cold or else hot enough to actually swim.

THE SCHOOL OF
WATER TREATMENT

When backpacking, your water sources will vary from beaver ponds to cool, free-flowing springs. And you never know where you're going to run into one of those little nasties that can make a backpacking trip your ultimate nightmare. So what exactly are you looking to remove? Most means of treating water are designed to kill or filter some or all of the following:

bacteria: Smaller than protozoans, bacteria can range in size from 0.2 microns to 10 microns. They cause problems ranging from food poisoning to typhoid fever.

cryptosporidium: Crypto, for short, is a tenacious bacteria. Unfortunately, no one knows for sure how prevalent this little bug is. It is found less frequently than *Giardia*, but is still out there in the wild. The only way to eliminate crypto is to boil your water, treat it with chlorine dioxide, or use a filter with a pore size no larger than 2 microns.

organic chemicals: Blame this one on your fellow human beings who created them. These contaminants are the result of industrial and agricultural pollution and include pesticides, herbicides, diesel fuel, fertilizers, and the run-off from strip mines—all of which are things with which you can come in contact even in the deepest of wilderness (not that there is much of that left). In general, watch out in areas that look like they have been farmed, logged, mined, or used industrially. Gee, that pretty much covers at least the Lower 48! And, if the water smells bad or is discolored, be extra wary.

protozoans: These hard-shelled, single-celled parasites or cysts are the largest of the water-borne microorganisms. They range in size from 2 to 15 microns and are the family to which the carrier of that infamous hiker disease, Beaver Fever, otherwise known as *Giardia lamblia*, belongs. Most filters and methods of chemical treatment will handle these.

viruses: The smallest of the small, viruses range in size from 0.0004 to 0.1 microns. They are probably the most dangerous of the waterborne monsters. The types of disease they carry, such as hepatitis, are enough to make the strongest backpacker want to hightail it to the nearest Hyatt. Fortunately, for those who are inclined, hepatitis vaccines are available, as well as vaccines for just about any viral agent you may encounter. And if you're still scared, buy the smallest micron-pore available. Also, the filter manufacturer SweetWater recommends combining chemical treatment with a filter. They sell the chlorine treatment ViralStop to be used in conjunction with a water filter for maxium safety.

TREATING WATER

Boiling your water is the easiest solution, particularly at dinnertime. At least one minute, and as many as three-to-five at higher altitudes, at a brisk boil will kill most of the bad things that inhabit outdoor water sources. But the problem is the time it takes to set up and boil the water. Who wants to boil water when they only want a quick drink? And who wants to take the time to boil water when they want to make miles? And finally, who wants to boil water on a blazingly hot day?

CHEMICAL TREATMENT

Iodine works, although it is not completely reliable against *Giardia*, but the taste? Potable Aqua or a similar product helps mitigate the taste of iodine, but without it, even powdered drinks barely mask it.

A fairly new option for chemical treatment is the use of chlorine dioxide, which is sold by the brand name Aqua Mira in the United States, and as the brand Pristine in Canada. Chlorine dioxide is a two-part solution. You mix drops from each of the two bottles together to form chlorine dioxide in five minutes. Add the mixture to a liter of water, and it is purified in about 30 minutes, depending on the water temperature and clarity.

The mix procedure is fairly easy and the treatment works well. Unlike iodine, Aqua Mira kills *Cryptosporidium*. But the big advantage of Aqua Mira for many hikers and backpackers is that it has practically no taste. No iodine taste, and even less chlorine taste than most city water. Some hikers even claim that it improves the taste of water along the Trail. Perhaps the best endorsement is that chlorine dioxide is the water treatment method used by clean-water guru Ryan Jordan.

Aqua Mira costs $14 for enough of the two-part solution to treat 114 liters of water—a cost of roughly 12 cents per liter of treated water. Even if you opt to carry a water filter, you will probably want to have Aqua Mira with you as a back up.

A new product recently developed by MSR is the MiOx purifier. This tiny (3.5 ounces and the size of a Maglight) water purifier is particularly useful in treating large quantities of water. It works by creating a powerful dose of mixed

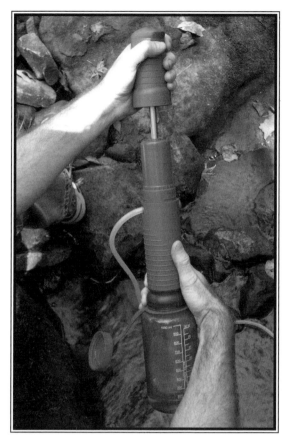

Purifying water with a Katadyn ceramic filter

oxidants (thus, MiOx) which is then added to untreated water, inactivating all viruses, bacteria, *Giardia*, and *Cryptosporidium* (which even iodine doesn't kill). And since the MiOx purifier needs only common camera batteries and salt to operate, it's maintenance-free.

While the MiOx system is not overly complicated, it does require a multistep process, which is explained fully in an accompanying handbook. It includes getting the mix right and using test strips to make sure the water is safe to drink (another plus). While using MiOx is an involved process, and, like other chemical treatments, takes time (a minimum of 20 minutes), it does deliver a high level of treatment and has no expiration date; as long as salt is available the unit is ready to purify water, time after time after time. Another benefit is that the treatment does not alter the taste of the water like chlorine and iodine do. This purifier makes more sense for use in a group—the pouring, stirring, mixing, and test-stripping seem worth it when you're purifying four gallons, less so when doing a single bottle of water. And, as with most treatments, you will need to prefilter water that has major particles in it. The MiOx system is also a bit on the expensive side—about $130.

ULTRAVIOLET LIGHT

Another pricey, but effective, option is the use of ultraviolet light. Without heat or chemicals, ultraviolet light destroys bacteria, protozoa, and viruses. This form of treatment is standard in bottle-water plants, but new to the backcountry. The Steri-pen is a hiker-friendly product, which treats a liter of water in 80 seconds.

Just insert the pen into the water bottle, push the button, and the electronics in the sterilizer determine the proper dose duration. The liquid level sensors ensure that the germicidal ultraviolet lamp is adequately immersed in the water, then microcomputer activates the lamp for the dose period of between 38 and 48 seconds. After less than a minute of gentle stirring the water is disinfected and ready to drink. At $150 per unit, the price per liter for 5,000 uses weighs in at about 23 cents per liter.

The battery-powered Steri-pen weights 8 ounces (with batteries) and is approximately 7 inches tall and 1.5 inches at its widest point. Steri-Pen uses four disposable or externally rechargeable AA batteries, which can be found virtually anywhere in the world. Alkaline batteries provide 20 to 40 treatments; 1800mAh NiMH rechargeable batteries provide about 100 treatments; and lithium batteries provide 130 to 140 treatments. One couple who thru-hiked using the Steri-pen noted that it took just five sets of lithium batteries for the whole thru-hike. Another solo hiker used just three sets of batteries for his hike.

WATER FILTERS

There are two important factors to weigh before deciding on a water filter—how easy and reliable the filter is to use and how effective the filter is.

We can tell you what you need to look for in a filter but, unfortunately, with the ever-changing technology and with something as important as a filter, you might need more than the manufacturer's guarantee that its filter will do the best job for you without failing when you need it the most. One means of evaluating filters is to visit a consumer Web site such as **www.epinions.com** or an online A.T. forum such as **www.whiteblaze.net.**

A filter's effectiveness is even tougher to judge, because we only have the manufacturer's word that the filter eliminates what it claims to eliminate. There are, as yet, no independent tests done on water filters to determine how they measure up to their claims. Basically, you just gotta take their word for it. One way to bolster your ability to make an informed choice is to do some independent research on water treatment. Visit manufacturer Web sites to learn basic facts. For the more hardcore seeker of truth, try out technical resources such as the Center for Biofilm Engineering's Web site at **www.erc.montana.edu,** and take a peek at the Center's for Disease Control and Prevention's site at **www.cdc.gov.**

One word of caution: Don't risk clogging that precious filter by filtering your cooking water. You've got to bring it to a boil anyway—just boil it for three minutes no matter what (this can include cooking time). You'll always be on the safe side, and not a single one of the little bad guys out there will survive a three-minute dip in a rolling boil. Just fill your cook pot with unfiltered water and set it on the stove.

Types of Filters

gravity feed filter: A great filter if you're not in a hurry. Water is scooped into a reservoir and then the filter is hung from a tree or overhang. While you wait (or tend to chores) the water trickles through the filter element into a receptacle—basically, a portable Brita filter.

pump filter: This filter uses a hand pump to suck water through an intake hose before passing it through the filter element and out through the outlet hose. Just stand over the stream (or pond or river, etc.) and pump away. These filters are faster and more efficient than gravity feed filters, and the better filters are fairly easy to pump. Because these filters require a lot of mechanical parts susceptible to breaking and clogging, always carry along a repair kit and extra parts.

straw/squeeze bottle filter: These are water bottles with a filter element fitted within the lid or the straw that runs into the bottle. It works by dipping the bottle in the water source to fill it and then sucking or squeezing to filter. The filter in this type tends to remove only the larger organisms although some bottles offer an iodine back-up system.

So now that you know about the different types of filters, you can learn that most of the filters on the market today use what is known as a *depth filter*. This means that the filter element has some depth to it that allows it time to capture the microorganisms. Depth filters can be cleaned by either scrubbing or backwashing (pumping the water backwards through the filter to release the clogged sediment). Surface filters are also used, but more rarely. These are essentially a single-layer filter that catches as catch can. The following are the different types of active ingredients used in both styles of filter.

Filter Elements

carbon: Carbon is often used with other filter materials to strain out organic chemicals like herbicides, pesticides, and chlorine. Carbon can also make bad-tasting water a little tastier.

ceramic: This porous material has lots of little nooks and crannies (kind of like an English muffin) to capture microorganisms. Ceramic filters last a long time and can be cleaned over and over again before they have to be replaced. The major drawback is that ceramic is fragile and will often crack in cold weather.

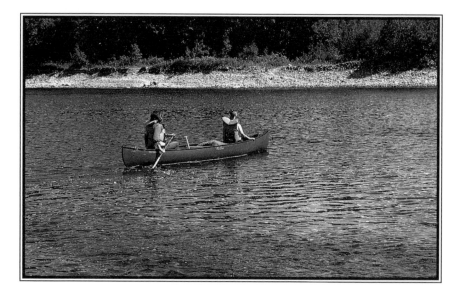

Victoria Logue taking the canoe ferry across Kennebec River in Maine

fiberglass or glass fiber: Long and slick, glass fibers can be molded into the intricate designs needed to catch microorganisms. While not as long-lasting as ceramic, fiberglass is less fragile and doesn't crack in cold weather.

proprietary: Yes, it's that secret code word that manufacturers use to mean, "we ain't tellin' what our filter uses." So, how and why these work, we don't know.

Another major feature to consider when purchasing a filter is the pore size. Pore size is the diameter of the openings in the filter element. Pore size determines how big a nasty has to be to get caught in the filter, which in turn determines the types of particles or microorganisms that are caught. To remove protozoans such as *Giardia*, the pore size must be 4 microns or smaller. But to remove bacteria, the pore size has to be at least 0.2 microns in size (big difference in the world of microns). And if you want to hear something really scary, some viruses can be as small as 0.0004 microns in size. The period at the end of this sentence is approximately 500 microns in size. Yikes! What does that mean? It means that no filter can effectively remove all types of viruses. On the other hand, the chances of consuming one of those micro-micro viruses is very slim. Even if you do consume an unfilterable virus, that does not mean you will automatically fall ill. Three factors—dose of the germ, virility of the germ, and your own immune status—combine to determine if the virus will make you sick. This is also true of all infectious microorganisms.

When picking out a filter, check for the "absolute" pore size as opposed to the "nominal" size. The absolute will tell you that the filter will not pass anything larger than that size. The nominal, on the other hand, only lets you know that a filter will remove most, but not all, particles larger than that size.

It is good idea to carry along a pre-filter that attaches to your filter's intake hose, or even a bandana to remove the really large particles that are greedily looking forward to clogging up your filter element.

Should your filter become clogged anyway, and at some point it probably will, carry along these items in your repair kit:

- **A scrubber sponge or toothbrush to clean the filter element.** Scrub the element once, rinse, and then scrub again. Check your manufacturer's suggestions first, though—some filters are not designed to be scrubbed.
- **Spare O-rings** to replace the ones that might break or crack and cause leaks. The manufacturer should be able to supply these.
- **A lubricant.** O-rings can dry out and ruin the seal on a filter. A tube of lubricant (also available from the manufacturer) can alleviate this problem. No lubricant? Use cooking oil or spit. Do not use petroleum-based products.
- **A bandana and a rubber band.** As mentioned above, a bandana used as a pre-filter can significantly increase the life of your filter. Secure it with the rubber band to free your hands for pumping or whatever.

For a rough estimate of how long you have until sunset, hold your hand out at arm's length and line your fingers up with the horizon. Each finger that you can fit between the horizon and the bottom of the sun represents about 15 minutes. If six fingers separate the sun and land, the sun should set in about one-and-a-half hours.

Chapter Four

Shelters and Tents

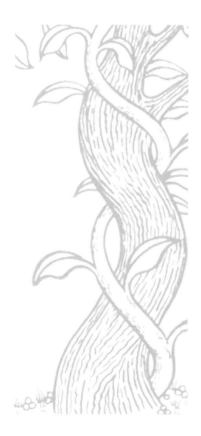

Though sleeping under the stars might be romantic in perfect conditions, the truth is conditions are rarely perfect. From rain and snow to mosquitoes and black flies, something is bound to come along and wreck your perfect evening. There is a reason that early man first found shelter in caves and quickly learned to design their own forms of shelter. Even the desert Bedouins carry protective tents as they travel across the desert. And that is why, when planning an overnight hike on the Appalachian Trail, be it one night or three-hundred and sixty-five, it is essential to plan for some sort of shelter. Many is the time we have gone to sleep under a starry sky only to be awakened by rain or snow.

SHELTERS

The chain of shelters and lean-tos along the length of the Appalachian Trail is a blessing to hikers. From Springer Mountain Shelter in Georgia to the lean-tos at Katahdin Stream Campground in Maine, the shelter system adds an important dimension to hiking the A.T.

A shelter is often a welcome sight at the end of a day's journey. In fact, it is not uncommon for hikers to be looking around every corner for the shelter that marks the day's last mile. A lean-to can be a dry place to rest or seek shelter for the night during a storm.

Unfortunately, finding an empty shelter during periods of peak use has become a rare occurrence, though you should find "room in the inn" if you arrive in the early afternoon. The later in the day you arrive at a shelter, the more likely it will be full. This is also a seasonal problem. For example, hiking in New Hampshire and Maine in August, you will find lots of fellow hikers. In Virginia's Shenandoah National Park, leaf-peepers fill the park during foliage season in late October. Some shelters have established camping areas around them, but check your guidebook for exact locations. Never count on staying in a shelter or even camping at one (some shelters do not allow tents nearby). It is possible that you might have to push on another couple of miles (sometimes in the dark) to find a decent camping spot after coming upon a full shelter with no available camping sites.

Shelters are generally free and available to all hikers on a first-come, first-served basis. Groups should take care not to monopolize the facilities and should yield to solo hikers and small groups. Some shelters that receive heavy use have caretakers to educate hikers on minimum-impact camping and proper use of Trail resources.

More than 260 three-sided shelters or lean-tos are located along the A.T., at various intervals (ranging from only 1 mile to more than 30, with an average of 9 miles). Designs vary, but typical features include:

- Raised wooden floors
- Overhanging roofs
- Room for 6 to 12 people

- Nearby privy and water source (usually a spring or stream, but may also be a pond or something else)
- Limited number of primitive campsites nearby (except where regulations prohibit it)

There is a good deal of variety in the design of shelters. Most are built of log, but some are made of stone, and a few of concrete. Only a handful of the original low-slung log shelters built in the 1930s remain; newer shelters tend to be more spacious and accommodate more hikers. Due to the finite number of potential sites for shelters, focus has increasingly been on renovating older shelters. Of particular concern in recent years has been creating designs that encourage hikers to prepare, eat, and store food away from sleeping areas to minimize human–animal interactions.

Nowhere is this trend more evident than in the Smokies. This park's shelter system, unique on the A.T., used to feature chain-link fences across the front of the shelter to keep the bears out. This led to hikers storing their food in the shelters, cooking inside, and creating conditions that led the bears to associate the shelters with food. The chain-link fences are being removed, the shelters renovated, and food-storage cables provided. Today, hikers are encouraged to eat and cook away from the shelters, and are required to hang their food and other "smellables" on cables provided for this purpose.

There are some shelters along the Appalachian Trail that charge a small fee. For example, in the White Mountains, the Appalachian Mountain Club maintains a series of tentsites, shelters, campsites, and huts (see *Preparing for Your First Hike,* page 173, for more on these). Tentsites have designated tenting areas with platforms or pads; shelters are either three- or four-sided structures; and campsites have a mixture of cabins and tent areas.

Caretakers are in residence at the following tentsites, shelters, and campsites in New Hampshire, and an overnight fee is charged:

Ethan Pond Campsite	Liberty Spring Campsite
Guyot Campsite	Nauman Tentsite
Imp Campsite	Speck Pond Campsite
Kinsman Pond Campsite	13 Falls Tentsite

The remaining tentsites, shelters, and campsites are available to backcountry travelers at no charge. These sites are available on a first-come, first-serve basis. Thru-hikers who wish to stay at any of AMC's facilities as paying guests will be offered the reduced club-member rate. Because fees and the groups that charge them can change annually, and because shelters may be relocated, it is best to check just prior to your trip.

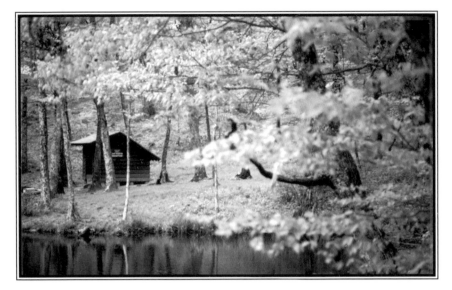

Punchbowl Shelter in central Virginia

Shelters in heavy-use areas often require a permit, registration, and/or fees. These include:

Great Smoky Mountains National Park (Tennessee and North Carolina)
Shenandoah National Park (Virginia)
White Mountain National Forest (New Hampshire)
Green Mountain National Forest (Vermont)
Baxter State Park (Maine)

More comprehensive information is available through the Appalachian Trail Conservancy in its regional maps and guidebooks. The most up-to-date information is available through the *Appalachian Trail Data Book* and *The Appalachian Trail Thru-hiker's Companion*, which are updated annually.

SHELTER EXCEPTIONS

In the Great Smoky Mountains National Park, shelter reservations and a permit are required, unless you begin your hike 50 miles outside of the park and plan to continue 50 miles beyond the park.

In Baxter State Park, a shelter known as the Birches is exclusively for use by I.A.T. hikers who have hiked at least 100 miles to reach the shelter. A.T. flip-floppers and southbounders are not allowed. The I.A.T. starts where the Appalachian Trail ends—one vertical mile straight up, on the summit of Katahdin in Baxter State Park. From Katahdin, the I.A.T. heads north through Maine, crosses briefly into New Brunswick, then turns east and traverses the length of Quebec's remote Chic Chok Mountains. The I.A.T. finishes at the eastern tip of Quebec's Gaspé peninsula, at Cape Gaspé, extending the A.T. another 687 miles. This is truly an "international" trail; the full name for this rugged, new footpath is the Sentier International des Appalaches/International Appalachian Trail, or S.I.A/I.A.T.

TRAIL REGISTERS

Zen-ish observations, diatribes on trail maintenance, exaltations of the natural world, and autobiographical ramblings are among the scribbles and scrawls found in trail registers. The writings left behind by hikers range from the monotonous to the brilliant, but they all give some idea of the types of people who spend time on the Trail.

Started as a safety measure to pinpoint the whereabouts of hikers, trail registers (usually spiral-bound notebooks) have become an important link in a vast communications network. Trail registers offer hikers the chance to make comments to those behind them, and to get to know, sometimes intimately, those ahead.

Along the same vein, "trail names" can become an important identifier even if you hike on the Trail only a few days a year. Trail names are the nicknames used by hikers to identify themselves in registers.

The Appalachian Trail Conservancy has a couple of requests regarding these unofficial trail registers. Profanity should not be used because families hike the Trail and read the registers; don't write anything you wouldn't want a secondgrader to read.

Also, refrain from berating trail maintainers' performance and the hiking styles of others. The trail maintainers do their monumental task on a volunteer basis, and without their important work the Trail wouldn't exist. As for hiking styles, any hiking style is correct if it suits the person using it. If someone hikes much faster than you, it doesn't mean that person is going too fast; it only means that he or she is doing more miles in a day than you care to do. The same goes for

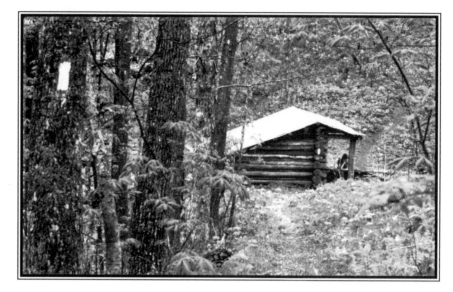

Spring Mountain Shelter near Hot Springs, North Carolina

those who hike fewer miles in a day. It's not a contest and there are no prizes, so the ATC asks that you keep your criticism of others to yourself.

With that said, remember how important others' entries can be to you. If you have something on your mind, don't be afraid to share it. After a tough day of slogging through the rain, a read through the register can be entertaining. On the other hand, entries that ramble on for more than a page often go unread.

To fulfill the registers' initial purpose of keeping tabs on hikers should an emergency occur, always give the date, the time of day, your name, and your trail name, and where you are headed next. This practice allowed me (Victoria) to be notified in New Hampshire within a few hours of my grandfather's death in Georgia. Needless to say, my family was grateful that I could be located so easily. It is also a good idea to make sure the folks back home know your trail name as this will help them find you in case of an emergency.

C A M P S I T E S

S helters may not be located where you are looking to spend the night. They may also be full. And let's face it—you don't always want to spend the night with whoever happens to drop in at a given shelter.

A.T. maintaining clubs have created some tentsites along the Trail. These designated campsites provide a flat, cleared place to pitch a tent, a water source, and occasionally a privy. Some heavy-use areas have one or more tent platforms to reduce the environmental impact.

Generally speaking, camping is restricted to designated campsites and shelters to concentrate hiker impacts where use is highest: in the Smokies, Maryland, New Jersey, New York, Connecticut, parts of the White Mountain National Forest, and Baxter State Park in Maine. Camping is prohibited in Harpers Ferry National Historical Park. Additionally, some other parks and forests also have specific restrictions or prohibitions pertaining to camping.

Camping wherever you can find a suitable site is allowed along much of the A.T., especially in the south. In some areas there may be restrictions. For example, in Shenandoah National Park, hikers are prohibited from camping within 50 yards of another camping party or a "no camping" post and must follow other guidelines. While on Pennsylvania Game Lands, hikers must camp within 200 feet of the Trail.

In many places along the A.T., the terrain is too rocky, too steep, too boggy, or the vegetation too thick for comfort. Locating a good campsite in a pristine area that does not involve disturbing the natural ground cover takes time and care. When you find a suitably flat and dry area (at least 200 feet from any water source) look for durable surfaces such as rock, gravel, or grassy areas that will be little affected by your camp.

Remember, "Good campsites are found not made." In other words, if you need to alter the site to make your tentsite comfortable, look elsewhere. If you happen upon an area that has received enough use to reduce it to bare ground, by all means use it. Once an area has reached this stage, the damage has already occurred and your stay will not impact it much further. Otherwise, look for resilient areas that show no signs of previous use and avoid areas where impact is just beginning and the site still has a chance to recover.

Before unpacking your tent or tarp, look for bird-nesting activity and other obvious signs of animals. Choose an area that seems safe, free of wildlife, and well suited to low-impact camping. Look overhead for large branches that seem ready to drop; there is a reason these are known as widowmakers. When choosing a place to cook your dinner, look for a large rock slab, a gravel area, or other equally durable space well away from your sleep area.

When breaking camp, naturalize and disguise the site by replacing any rocks or sticks you moved so that those who follow will be less likely to choose the site. Recover scuffed up areas with leaf litter or pine needles. Fluff up matted grass and make the place look less like a campsite. Research has shown that as few as five nights of camping use in a year can permanently impact vegetation. This creates a site that is still obvious a year later.

TENTS

Almost any hiker you speak to can tell you of a time they were glad they had their tent. They could also tell you of a time they cursed it. Tents have their advantages over tarps and over sleeping under the stars. It all depends on how much discomfort you're willing to withstand. And there are some parts of this country (and this world) where a tent is an absolute necessity just to separate the predators from the prey!

Strictly speaking, a large piece of plastic and some rope is all it takes. When asked what type of tent they prefer, backpackers will give a range of answers. From tarps to roomy dome tents (costing from $10 up for a tarp or tent, to tents costing more than $500), hikers will tell you that their tarp or tent has proven adequate.

For most A.T. hikers, a tent is a safeguard for staying dry on a rainy night, especially between shelters or when shelters are full. Tents keep out the rain and bugs, they are warm on cold nights because your body temperature warms the tent (sometimes by as much as ten degrees), and the tent itself dulls the force of the wind. When it's cold, wet, and buggy, tents are invaluable.

Important Features of Tents

SHAPE

Backpacking tents are designed in a variety of shapes, each with their own benefits and drawbacks.

A-FRAME: This classic shape is also known as the pup tent. Roomy and easy to set-up, A-frames tend to be stable except in the wind. They are usually inexpensive but they are rarely self-supporting, and many models have a support pole in the middle of the entrance, making getting in and out a little inconvenient.

MODIFIED A-FRAME: This is an A-frame with a center hoop pole, ridgeline pole, and/or curved end poles that allow for a lot more space on the inside as well as more structural stability. Some of the modified A-frames are free standing—that is, they don't require stakes to set them up.

DOME: The dome is probably the most popular backpacking tent, because it solves the limitations of the A-frame. Free-standing, roomy, stable, and taut in the wind, the dome also offers plenty of head and elbow room and maximum space for its weight. Consequently, its price runs a bit higher than the A-frame. Domes tend to be a bit heavier as well, and some dome tents do not fit easily into a pack. While they come in a variety of shapes and sizes with numerous configurations of poles, all domes are based on a geodesic design. Because of this, ventilation is poorer than in an A-frame, as there is not an obvious side in which to place a door and the floor plan is often a little odd.

A note from experience—dome tents are stable in the wind only if there is something inside them weighing them down. They make great kites if left empty on a windy day, especially if the door is open.

PYRAMID OR TEEPEE: The pyramid or teepee typically consists of a waterproof rainfly that drapes over a single pole (or walking stick) and stakes out to create a cone-shaped shelter. Some pyramid tents come with detachable floors. These are quite easy to set up and are generally lighter than other tents. Note that they provide little protection against bugs and are reliant on how well you can stake them.

TUNNEL OR HOOP: The tunnel tent is gaining in popularity because of the relation of floor space to the overall size (and weight) of the tent. Much lighter and more compact than other tents because of the "covered wagon," two-hoop design, tunnels are rarely free-standing and must be pitched in the right position to provide optimum stability in wind. Sleeping in an unstaked tunnel tent is similar to bedding down in a bivy sack—it keeps you out of the elements. Some of the newer models offer a third or middle hoop and numerous guy points to improve their stability.

ULTRALIGHT OR BIVY: A bivy (short for bivouac) is the barest minimum of tent in the tunnel design. The lightest and most compact of tents, the ultralight or bivy is not for the claustrophobic. As a matter of fact, some people classify the bivy sack as a sleeping bag rather than a tent.

Dome tents and some modified A-frames do not require that you stake them down to keep them from collapsing once you've pitched the poles. Not having to stake down your tent makes relocating, cleaning, and drying your tent much easier. But, if it is windy out, you'll want to stake it down anyway.

Single-wall construction means only that the tent does not have a rainfly. These tents are usually made of a fabric that is both waterproof and breathable. Because they are made of high-tech materials, they are often more expensive. But, they are also lighter and easier to pitch. While the walls are designed to vent moist air while keep the inclement weather at bay, most are susceptible to condensation in all but the driest of conditions. Seam sealing is a must.

WEIGHT

When you are making your tent wish list, remember that you will have to carry the tent. When questioned, most hikers say that the weight of a tent is its most important feature, leading a few to purchase a tarp and sleep screen.

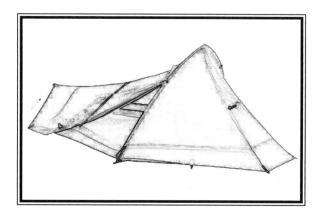

Waypoint by Mountain Hardwear

Carrying more tent than the trip calls for can be almost as much of a mistake as not having an adequate tent. As a rule of thumb, try not to carry more than four pounds of tent per person (three pounds is better). If two people are splitting the load, you will be able to carry a roomier tent. Having one person carry the poles and fly while the other carries the rest is one way to split it up. Another would be for one person to carry all the tent and the other person to carry the cooking gear and more food.

ROOM/CAPACITY

The second most important thing to look for in a tent is roominess. Are you tall? Is there enough room to stretch out to your full length? What about headroom? Do you have enough room to sit up comfortably if you so desire? Decide how much room is important to you before purchasing a tent. Also, will you be cooking inside your tent? On cold mornings, it isn't unusual to see steam rising from beneath the vestibules of tents as hikers heat water for coffee and oatmeal. If you think this is a possibility (something we never planned on but ended up doing countless times), make sure the vestibule has enough space beneath it so that it won't ignite. Whenever possible, place a flat rock beneath your stove for further insurance.

If a tent claims it holds one to two people, it means exactly. Two people will be a tight fit without gear, one person will fit with gear. Keep that in mind when considering how much you want your tent to hold.

VENTILATION/FLOOR SPACE/LAYOUT

Ventilation is another important tent feature. On hot, buggy nights there is nothing worse than being stifled in a poorly ventilated tent. Many tents these days offer plenty of no-see-um netting for cross ventilation as well as protection from bugs. If you are planning only cold-weather camping, this feature won't be necessary. On the other hand, if you intend to hike in every season, a good tent fly will compensate in cold weather for the extra ventilation needed in hot weather.

There are several tent floor space/layout options:

HEXAGONAL: This is the most common shape for dome tents. While it supplies enough room next to your elbows for assorted items, it isn't exactly designed for the very tall.

RECTANGULAR: Most A-frames and some domes have a rectangular shape. This limits floor space but allows the tall to stretch out without worry about hitting either end of the tent.

SQUARE: This type of floor plan is most often found in three- or four-person tents where the hikers are stacked side by side.

MISCELLANEOUS GEOMETRIC SHAPES: These are trapezoidal or otherwise-unusually-shaped tents that feature odd corners for stowing gear.

USAGE

Tents are available in a number of different styles that allow you to choose a make and model specific to how and when you intend to do the majority of your A.T. backpacking:

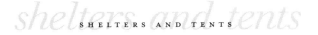

THREE-SEASON: These tents feature screened canopies and full rainflies with enough ventilation for muggy summer nights and the option for enough cover in the spring and fall to ward off late and early winter chills. Most of these tents come with two to four poles and a vestibule and offer enough room for two hikers. See *Winter Backpacking* (page 191) for a description of four-season tents.

SUMMER/SCREEN: These ultralight tents are mostly yards of mesh with a bare minimum for a rainfly. With only one or two poles, these tents seem to capture even the faintest breeze on even the hottest of nights but are not made for cool weather.

CONVERTIBLE: This hybrid is versatile because it comes with a number of pole, window, vestibule, and/or rainfly options. In the summer, you can leave a pole or full vestibule at home to carry less weight and unzip the window panels for more ventilation. When it is cold out, carry along the extra pole for added stability and the full vestibule to allow for more storage space and then zip the windows to increase the warmth inside the tent.

MOUNTAINEERING/HIGH ALTITUDE: These tents feature full coverage rainflies and are made from heavy-duty materials. They are extremely stable as they have been designed to withstand the notoriously unpredictable weather of high mountains. Most of these tents have four or more poles along with a large vestibule. Because they are made for high altitudes, they tend to be heavier and more expensive than other tents and offer less ventilation.

TENT MATERIALS

Most backpacking tents are made of a strong but lightweight nylon taffeta or ripstop nylon, which weighs approximately two ounces per square yard. The floor and flys are usually coated with urethane or another moisture-repellent substance to prevent moisture from passing through. Although the body of the tent is often left uncovered to increase the transfer of respiration and perspiration through the tent's walls, it is not unusual to wake up in a damp tent. We have found that moisture often gathers beneath our sleeping pads. The more water resistant and "breathable" the material (like Gore-Tex), the drier you'll be but the more expensive the tent will be.

TENT POLES

In the past few years, tent poles have evolved from unyielding steel to flexible, shock-corded, aluminum poles. Pole segments are threaded over elastic (shock) cord that allows the user to merely snap the poles into shape rather than piece them together. When dismantling the tent, the segments are pulled apart and folded compactly.

There is still some controversy as to whether fiberglass is superior to aluminum as a tent-pole material. Fiberglass is less expensive and more flexible than aluminum. It does not require pre-bending or any special attachments. It also provides a better packing size when folded. Its major drawback is that it weathers easier than aluminum and can break. Unlike aluminum, which can be splinted when it breaks (although it is more likely to bend), fiberglass breaks into clean splinters and must be replaced. Durability is one of aluminum's main advantages along with the fact that it is easily replaced.

Today, some tentmakers offer high-strength aluminum poles and even more expensive but stronger carbon-fiber poles.

WORKMANSHIP

Although any tent may be adequate for your needs, you may want to consider how long you would like your tent to last. Good workmanship means a long-lasting relationship with your tent. A well-made tent should have lap-felled seams around the floor seam. Lap-felled seams (like the seams on the sides of your Levis) provide extra strength because they are actually four layers of interlocking fabric joined by a double row of stitching. On uncoated nylon tents, check for taped seams. Because nylon tends to unravel, taping or hiding the end of the fabric behind the seam with another piece of fabric will stop or stall this process. Finally, make sure that all stress points are reinforced either with extra stitching or bar tacking. Tug at the material to make sure the load is equally distributed across the reinforcement. Unequal distribution can cause premature wear on your tent.

WATERPROOFING

Hikers agree that waterproofing is an important feature to consider. There is nothing more miserable than sleeping in a wet tent. The better the material (Gore-Tex is probably the gold standard, but treated nylon is most common), the more likely you are to sleep dry. But there are some days that it rains so hard that no matter how good your tent is, you're going to get wet. It may rain for days on end or you may not have the time to spare to dry your tent. As long as your sleeping bag is dry, you can sleep warmly, if not entirely comfortably, in a damp tent.

To keep your tent as dry as possible, it is important to seal its seams. Although parts of the tent are coated, the needle holes in the seams will allow water to enter your tent. Buy some sealer (available at most outdoors stores) and follow the directions. Then seal them again. Depending on how much you use your tent, the sealer can last up to two years. If you use your tent a lot, seal the seams more often. On an extended backpacking trip (five months or more), it may be necessary to reseal your seams at least once, if not several times.

SETUP

You will also want to consider how easily a tent can be set up and taken down—important when it comes to pitching a tent in the rain or wind. Practice setting up your tent before you begin a long hike. The time saved by knowing your tent could mean the difference between soggy and dry clothes.

COLOR

While color is a matter of personal preference, there are valid reasons why you may choose one over the other. Bright, neon-like colors are useful in search-and-rescue conditions because the blinding material will stand out against the snow, the green and brown of the woods, or the sand in the desert. For the same reason, bright colors along the A.T. might be annoying to other backpackers, causing a visual disturbance in the wilderness.

If your tent is pale green or blue, the bright sunlight filtered through your tent will form a soft light inside. On rainy or overcast days, the light inside your tent could be slightly depressing. These colors are also a bit more inconspicuous in the backcountry.

Orange and yellow fabric are great in foul weather because they produce a brighter light inside your tent. Grey, light grey, white, and tan are popular colors now and are also pleasing to the eye inside and outside the tent. Blue and gold are also used in many tents.

GROUND CLOTHS

A plastic ground cloth, cut to fit under the bottom of your tent, may not completely protect the tent from the damp (or wet), but it helps. Ground cloths come in handy especially when setting your tent up on ground that has been wet for days. They also reduce the wear and tear on the floor of your tent.

If the ground cloth is larger than your tent, you are likely to wake up in the middle of a rainy night sitting in the puddle that has formed beneath your tent. By cutting it to within an inch of your tent's width and length, you'll wake up much drier. Another possibility (rather than setting your tent on top of the ground cloth) is putting the ground cloth inside the tent. The bottom of your tent gets wet, but the equipment and people inside stay drier.

Plastic remains a popular groundcloth material, but the better option today is to use a house wrap, such as Tyvek, which is available from a hardware store. The insulative house wrap makes a more durable, yet still lightweight ground cloth.

Pitching Tents in the Wind, Snow, and Rain

Before embarking on any backpacking trip, you should know your tent (and all your other equipment for that matter) backwards and forwards. Set it up in your backyard (or if that is impossible, your living room) over and over again until you can do it in your sleep. This will be invaluable once you're in the backcountry and setting up your tent in a downpour or in a raging wind.

At the end of the day, when you want nothing more than to crawl into your sleeping bag and drift off to sleep, you must first set up your tent. If there is a knock-you-off-your-feet wind blowing, first visualize the steps for setting up your tent. If you get panicky and insert the wrong pole into the wrong sleeve, it will take twice as long to pitch.

Before unrolling your tent, have the poles, stakes, and whatever else you need to set up ready. As you slowly unroll your tent, stake it to the ground if it is not a freestanding tent. If you have a friend, have her or him lay down inside the unpitched tent to take some chaos out of the process. If it is freestanding, place heavy objects on the tent floor to keep it from blowing away.

Once pegged or weighted to the ground, insert poles windward side first. This sounds easier than it is, but with a little determination and imagination your tent will soon be up. If it is a freestanding tent, throw your pack inside to weigh the tent down until you get in. If it is a pegged tent, make sure none of the stakes threaten to pull loose.

If you plan a backpacking trip in the snow, make sure that you have pegs that will hold in both soft and hard snow. Most outdoors stores offer special anchors and pegs for snow camping. You may want to purchase a full-time replacement for the spindly pegs that come with your tent. Some of the heavy-duty options available are T-stakes, I-beams, half-moons, and corkscrews. The salesman at your outdoors store will be able to tell you which stake best suits your purpose. Making sure your tent is securely pegged is important when setting up your tent on snow. Before you can set up your tent, you must first stamp down the snow, including an area for you to walk around while pitching your tent, and create a broad area for the entrance and troughs for the guylines, if you need them.

To keep your tent as dry as possible, make sure that you rid yourself of as much snow as possible before climbing in. A large garbage bag outside the entrance to your tent can work as a waterproof doormat.

If you intend to camp in extreme snow conditions, you will need either a snow shovel or something that can be used as a shovel such as a snowshoe. If your tent is buried in the snow, death as a result of oxygen deprivation or carbon monoxide poisoning is possible. If snow keeps falling for more than a day, take down your tent and rebuild your platform by shoveling snow onto the packed area and re-stamping. Finally, repitch your tent.

Pitching your tent in the rain is merely a matter of speed. It all comes down to how quickly you wish to get out of the rain. The faster you set up your tent, the quicker you can get dry. Getting the rainproof fly on as quickly as possible is very important. When taking down your tent in the rain, you may be able to do most of the work beneath the fly, keeping the tent a bit drier.

TAKING CARE OF YOUR TENT

Never store your tent when it is damp. Make sure it is thoroughly dry if you are going to put it up for more than a day. Otherwise, next time you pull it out of its stuff sack, you're bound to find it spotted with mold and mildew. It is important to make sure that even the seams are dry and that all the dirt has been cleaned from the stakes, poles, and bottom of the tent. Also, to avoid damaging your tent, carry your poles and pegs in a separate stuff sack.

When packing your tent, stuff it rather than rolling or folding it. If the fabric is stressed at the same points every time, it will eventually crack and peel. Never store your tent in your car or its trunk. Cars can become hot as a furnace, and those high temperatures can damage the coating on the tent's material.

To clean your tent, use a damp sponge and mild soap. Set up the tent before wiping it down and then let it air dry. If your tent is smeared with pitch or grease, use a bit of kerosene to remove it. Never machine-wash your tent.

Never leave your tent set up in the sun for long periods of time. If you are camping in one spot for several days, cover your tent with its fly during the day to protect it from the sun's ultraviolet rays, which can damage the nylon material. A fly is less susceptible to the sun's damage and can be replaced at less expense than the tent.

Keep your tent poles clean to avoid corrosion of the metal. A silicone lubricant occasionally applied to joints will help protect your poles and keep them in good working order. Also apply the silicone to your tent's zippers to keep them working smoothly when it's freezing outside.

Repair kits for your tent are very helpful and are available from most outdoor retailers. There are several kits available, but the best, in my opinion, is made by Outdoor Research. This inexpensive kit contains: adhesive-backed ripstop nylon and adhesive-backed taffeta fabric to repair holes in tent and fly fabric; mosquito netting; needle and thread to repair holes in no-see-um fabric; an aluminum splint and duct tape to repair broken tent poles; and braided Dacron utility cord in case you need to jerry-rig a guyline, tent-peg loop, etc. A small tent-repair kit should take care of most of the mishaps that can occur to a tent on a backpacking trip (unless you set the tent ablaze with your cooking stove or campfire).

TARPS

Hikers interested in cutting pack weight need to cast a critical eye on their tents. After all, even a lightweight tent is a heavy shelter when trying to break into the ultralight backpacking. When pitched properly, tarps are more weather tight than you would imagine. They can even be warmer than tents since they do not promote the build up of condensation that saps a sleeping hiker's body heat.

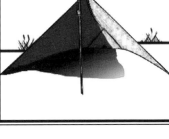

The Cave 1 by GoLite

Tarps do have their disadvantages, especially the open invitation to bugs. Escaping from bugs is no joke, and most tarp users agree that a sleep screen is indispensable when the mosquitoes, deerflies, and black flies arrive to torture innocent hikers.

HAMMOCKS

If you are tired of rocks and roots disturbing your sleep, a hammock may be your best option. Forget the primitive-style hammocks Gilligan and the Skipper slept in on TV—hammocks have gone high-tech. And before you go knocking hammocks, make sure you know who you are speaking with first, as hammockers have quite a loyal cult following.

One popular example is the Hennessy Hammock, which is a sleep system offering shelter with your hammock. From just a hair under two pounds, these hammocks cut pack weight while enhancing sleep comfort. The entrance is through the bottom of the hammock, leaving no openings for rain and bugs. Your body weight keeps the doorway closed until you are ready to get out. If no trees are available, they become a workable bivy sack.

Other models of hiking hammocks include The Clark Jungle Hammock and Crazy Crib's Crazy Crib LEX.

SLEEPING UNDER THE STARS

If you have a wonderfully comfortable sleeping bag, sleeping out under the stars is a viable option as long as you have a tent or tarp as backup, especially in the mountains, where weather can change in an instant.

Advantages to sleeping outdoors (other than not having to set up a tent or tarp) are mainly aesthetic: falling asleep under the stars and waking up to a sunrise. With your head outdoors, you can fall asleep and wake up to the wonders of nature.

As long as you're in a relatively safe area, the weather is good, and your sleeping bag warm, there is no reason not to enjoy a night under the stars. Just remember to have your food and other "smellables" hanging safely away from camp. As long as you use a little common sense, fresh-air camping is a pleasant experience.

If you're searching for the warmest site to pitch your tent, try a spot 15 feet higher than a stream, lake, or meadow. The slight change in elevation really can result in 15 more degrees. Also, the south and west sides of trees and rocks soak up sunshine during the day and radiate heat at night. Finally, cold air flows down a valley at night, close to the ground, and into the mouths of sleeping bags! Face yours downstream, if possible; it will be a lot warmer.

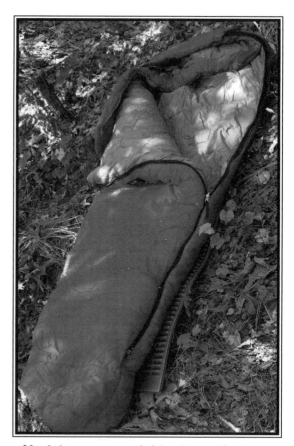

No shelter or tent needed in nice weather

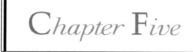

Chapter Five

Backpacks

In 2004, the Outdoor Industry Foundation (OIF) reported that 28 percent of the U.S. population considered themselves backpackers or hikers. Among outdoor activities monitored by the OIF, backpacking and hiking shared the top spot, in terms of sheer numbers. That's a lot of folks; that's a lot of backpacks, too, and the choices can be daunting.

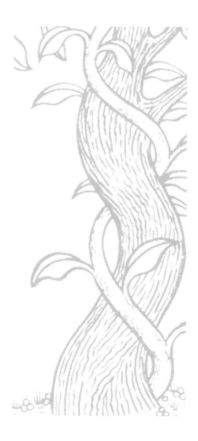

Backpacks are what separate the casual walker from the serious trekker. With just a daypack, you can spend hours or an entire day enjoying what the Appalachian Trail has to offer, knowing that home is waiting. Or you might drive up to a campsite and spend the night with nature, but the car and civilization is always close at hand. However, once you sling a backpack on your back, that changes. You intend to stay in the woods, often far from roads. When you carry everything you need, when you decide to depend on your own knowledge and the resources that will fit in a pack, you encounter an entirely new perspective on life. Perhaps that's why so many people have discovered a passion for backpacking. There is something about being completely self-sufficient, something about being one-on-one with the outdoors, that can't be beat.

Of those people who identify themselves as backpackers, the OIF discovered some interesting attitudes that backpackers share. Eighty-eight percent say that they enjoy the feeling of accomplishment as well as the feeling of escape from the mundane pressures of everyday life, that backpacking gives them. Over 75 percent of backpackers and hikers feel that the sport keeps them young, that it allows them to connect with themselves and with family members. That's a lot of positive energy.

But before you reach this state of self-sufficiency and truly discover the joys of backpacking, you're going to need a backpack. What kind do you need? Well, that depends . . . .

EXTERNAL VERSUS INTERNAL FRAME

While internal-frame packs are the current pack of choice with A.T. long-distance hikers, each pack style has pros and cons to consider. Here are the basic differences between the two: the external frame is designed to distribute weight equally and has a high center of gravity (perfect for established trails), while the internal-frame pack is designed to ease off-trail travel and has a lower center of gravity (popular for off-trail hiking and mountaineering).

In terms of keeping cool, external frames are superior. They also have more pockets in which to stow and organize items. The packs don't sag, and they are built to carry heavier loads more comfortably. Externals also tend to be less expensive than internals. On the other hand, internals provide better balance and pass through rocks, trees, and underbrush easier because they have fewer outside bulges and pockets.

Hip Belts

One common, and critical, area the two packs styles have in common is the hip belt. The hip belt carries the bulk of the weight, so that a properly fitted pack allows you to drop one shoulder out of its strap without a significant change in weight distribution. The hip belt should be padded, well built, and snug-fitting. Many companies offer optional hip belts that are larger or smaller than the standard adjustable hip belt. If you're planning a long-distance hike, remember that weight loss may cause the hip belt that fit you when you began to not fit you later in your trip.

Hip belts are also prone to breaking because of the amount of stress they receive. Because the internal frame's hip belt is usually an integral part of the pack, the entire pack often needs to be returned to fix it, though some pack manufacturers are beginning to make interchangeable parts for internal-frame packs. If a hip belt breaks on externals, you can usually remove the hip belts for repair. Manufacturers are usually great about replacing them free of charge. Keep the manufacturer's telephone number handy in case you need to order another hip belt or have one replaced.

Here are some more things to think about when considering a pack.

External Frame

External-frame packs come in top-loading, front-loading, and combination models. A top-loading pack works like a duffle bag attached to a frame, whereas front-loading packs give you easy access to your gear. Most manufacturers design their external packs with both a top-loaded and front-loaded section as well as front and side pockets.

Manufacturers of external-frame packs boast that the frame keeps the pack away from your body and thus is cooler in the summer. A good external-frame pack will have a mesh backband that will allow for circulation of air. This band should be tight and adjusted for your comfort.

Features to look for in an external-frame pack include:

- A welded tubular frame, preferably of a lightweight and strong material such as aluminum or molded plastic
- A coated nylon pack cloth (although not waterproof, it is water resistant—a pack cover is needed to waterproof your pack)
- Thick, padded shoulder straps

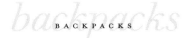

🌿 A mesh backband to allow air to circulate between your back and the pack

🌿 A thick, foam hipbelt with an easy-release buckle

🌿 Outside pockets on the pack bag

TIPS FOR FITTING AN EXTERNAL FRAME

🍃 When fitting your pack make sure that the shoulder straps are level with or an inch or two above the shoulders.

🍃 The mesh backband should fit snugly, but comfortably, against your back, and the hip belt should ride on your pelvis.

🍃 Adjust the hip belt up or down along the frame to prevent the lower end of the frame from making contact with your lower back.

🍃 Shoulder straps should not pinch your neck nor should they slide off your shoulders. Mounted too high, they put too much weight on your shoulders; too low, on your hips.

🍃 If the pack comes with load-lifters, they should join the frame at ear level and attach to the shoulder straps over your collarbone. Weight can be distributed from shoulders to hips with these straps.

🍃 A sternum strap will help hold the pack more closely to your back.

🍃 Accessory features in packs include ice-axe loops, crampon patches, ski holders, accessory pockets, and camera rings. On some packs you will find that these features are standard rather than optional.

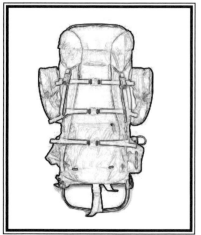

External frame
(JanSport Carson)

INTERNAL FRAME

Victoria had an agonizing time climbing through Maine's Mahoosuc Notch with her external-frame pack. The 0.9-mile stretch requires squeezing in and out, over and under endless tumbled boulders. Her external frame continually threw her off-balance, leaving her quaking in her boots and near tears. And every time she fell, she banged her head on the frame. At that moment, she would have done anything for an internal frame. Internal frames are designed to alleviate the problems

Victoria had in Maine. Because they hug your body and have a lower center of gravity (internal-frame packs are equipped with harnesses, straps, and other adjustments so that the pack may be form-fitted to each wearer), they enhance balance and allow more upper-body mobility and flexibility.

Most internal-frame packs are top-loading—the pack has a big top opening into which you dump what will fit, pack it down, and load some more. Okay, you're not really supposed to do it that way. For a top-loading pack, you need to be very organized. That way, not only do you know where all your stuff is, exactly, but you can also more evenly distribute the weight. Many top-loaders have extension tubes (basically a collar that extends up) to pro-

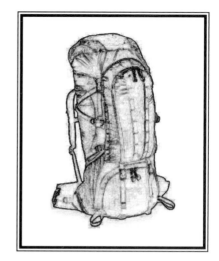

Internal frame
(Gregory Palisade)

vide additional volume with a floating lid to cover it all. With no zippers or a zipper only around the sleeping bag compartment, internal-frame packs are more water-resistant than externals.

However, there are more options out there. Panel-loading internal frame packs have one or more zippers on the front so you don't have to dig through all your stuff to get at whatever is on the bottom of the pack. Having more zippers, though, can make the pack harder to load due to the strain you create on zippers by overstuffing. Zippers also decrease a pack's overall resistance to water. If you do go for a panel-loader, make sure the zippers are really tough and there are at least one or two compression straps over the zippers to relieve some of the pressure (not to mention to hold things together should a zipper burst).

Hybrid-loading packs offer the best of both worlds because you can load from the top but you can also unzip to remove something near the bottom without unpacking everything. Once again, though, make sure the zippers are tough and that there is compression-strap backup.

There are two basic designs that make up the internal frame—parallel or X-shaped, depending on how the aluminum bars are sewn inside the packbag. These bars are custom bent to fit the curve of your back, then slid back into place. The internal frame is then fitted to your body by a number of straps attached to the packbag.

Things to look for in an internal frame include:

- Contoured aluminum stays to help distribute weight to your hips
- Thick, padded shoulder straps and hip belt
- A lumbar pad that will help support a heavy load and enhance ventilation
- Compression straps to keep smaller loads from shifting
- A reinforced bottom to resist abrasion
- A lot of lash points and loops to carry gear outside the pack
- A slim profile with either outside or add-on pockets
- Cinch straps at the shoulder and waist to keep the load close to your back

TIPS FOR FITTING AN INTERNAL FRAME

- Once the hip belt is fastened, make sure that the pack's stays protrude two to four inches above your shoulders. If the stays are outside this range, look for a pack that has a longer or shorter torso, respectively.

- If the padded ends of the hip belt overlap in front, the belt is too big. If they rub your belly, you'll need a larger belt.

- The pack fits you in the shoulders if the shoulder straps join the pack about two inches below the tops of your shoulders. The lower ends of the straps should be a hand's width below your armpits.

- Load-lifter straps should join your frame at ear level to comfortably divert pressure to the front of your shoulders. The buckles for these straps should be positioned over your collarbone. Weight can be distributed from waist to shoulders with these straps, and you should vary the position as you hike for the most comfort.

- If the pack hugs your back like a child holding on for a piggyback ride, you have a proper fit.

- If the waist belt is distorted by the way you cinched your stabilizing belts, the pack needs readjustment. Always make sure the pack is cinched tightly.

MORE PACK CONSIDERATIONS

PACK CAPACITY

Regardless of whether you choose an internal- or external-frame backpack, when looking for an appropriate pack you need to know how long you plan to be on the Trail. Generally, the longer you will travel, the larger the pack you will need. This isn't a hard-and-fast rule, however. Some advanced backpackers have learned to make due with a minimal amount of equipment. (This style of backpacking is often called fastpacking.) Nevertheless, here are some guidelines for the average hiker. Keep in mind that an internal pack will need about 1,000 cubic inches more space than externals, because sleeping bags are stuffed inside internals.

2,500 TO 3,000 CUBIC INCHES: This pack will handle the minimum needed for a warm-weather overnighter as long as you have a partner to share the task of carrying a small tent, cooking gear, and stove. This could also be a heavy-duty daypack. This type of pack has become especially popular with hikers who like to force themselves to carry less. The only drawback is that you can't carry enough gear for cold-weather hiking.

3,000 TO 4,000 CUBIC INCHES: This is the perfect pack for three-season weekend trips when you're carrying warm clothing and, once again, sharing gear. If you keep it simple, you can make a slightly longer trip with a pack this size. Due in part to the ultralight trend, this is the pack size of choice among most A.T. thru-hikers today.

4,000 TO 6,000 CUBIC INCHES: For those not inclined to make the philosophical leap toward ultralight gear, this is the perfect size pack for nearly all backpacking trips. You can head out for a weekend (alone or with a partner) or take off for a five-month trek on the A.T., if you like. This pack will handle a big load with ease.

6,000-PLUS CUBIC INCHES: Too large for most purposes, this pack is big enough for all the gear you'll need for a winter camping trip when it is cold and snowy, for a long expedition, or if you're the main load-bearer for a family outing.

Keep in mind that manufacturers have different ways of measuring the volume of their packs, and that a pack with 3,000 cubic inches may be slightly larger or smaller than another, though the difference is seldom, if ever, critical.

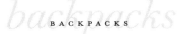

Pack Construction

Put some mileage on your pack and soon it will begin wearing out. The frame, seams, and zippers are especially subject to wear. Frank had a pack whose frame literally exploded off his back when it finally died. Victoria lost an adjustment strap on her hipbelt, a relatively minor inconvenience compared to the number of miles she put on that pack.

When purchasing a pack, check your pack frame (if you buy an external) for sturdiness and clean welds. Check the seams for even stitching and reinforcements, especially at the stress points. Make sure that there is sufficient room between the stitching and the edge of the seam and fabric because this is a likely place for it to separate. Feel free to tug and pull on the pack as much as you like— better to have it fall apart in the store than on your first trip out hiking. Buy a pack with heavy zippers. They are more durable. Also, if it is a front-loading pack, make sure there are compression straps to take the pressure off the zippers once loaded.

Pack Features

Even after deciding between internal, external, or a hybrid, the amount of features available on contemporary packs can be overwhelming. The following features are ones you will find on a wide range of backpacks:

ADJUSTABLE TORSO LENGTH: Some packs feature shoulder straps that move up and down to accommodate varying torso lengths. If the pack doesn't fit you right off the rack, this can be a great perk, because it allows you to adjust for a perfect fit. Make sure, if you go for this feature, that you know whether the pack has interchangeable suspension components or a fixed suspension. You'll have less adjustability with a fixed suspension but a more stable ride. Because the shoulder straps on an adjustable frame aren't locked into the frame, the harness can become wobbly when fully loaded.

DIVIDER BETWEEN MAIN COMPARTMENT AND SLEEPING-BAG COMPARTMENT: This feature allows you to remove the sleeping bag separately from the rest of the gear in the bag. Some packs have a removable divider as well.

DAYPACK CONVERSION: A removable lid or pocket can be used as a daypack or fanny pack.

HYDRATION BLADDER AND FEEDER TUBE: If you would rather suck water from a tube than stop and pull out a bottle, this pack option is for you. Packs that come with a "hydration system" usually consist of a bladder, a bladder sleeve or pocket, a feeder tube, and a slot for the tube to exit the pack.

INTERCHANGEABLE SUSPENSION PARTS: This system offers interchangeable shoulder straps and hipbelts to offer a more personalized fit.

SHOVEL POCKET: Once a feature for the cross-country skier's snow shovel, this pocket is now offered by some manufacturers as a convenient place to store rain gear or a jacket.

SPINDRIFT COLLAR: This is similar to a turtleneck on a shirt. Basically, the bag extends or stretches to contain gear that can't be fitted into the main compartment of the pack. They are particularly useful if you have a floating top lid. They also help keep out rain, snow, and dirt.

WATER-BOTTLE HOLSTERS: These are small pockets designed to hold your water bottle within easy reach.

WOMEN'S COMPONENTS: This is an interchangeable suspension system designed with women in mind. It helps conform a man's pack to a woman's body.

WOMEN'S MODEL BACKPACK: Some manufacturers came up with the radical idea that women might actually appreciate a pack designed with the female form in mind. These packs typically feature narrower shoulder straps, smaller hip belts, and shorter torsos. Imagine! Believe it or not, not all manufacturers offer women's packs, and those who do seldom offer more than a single model. Lowe offers the most options, with 9 women packs out of a stable of about 25. Maybe that's why Victoria loves her Lowe Sirocco.

PACK COVERS

Although all backpacks are made of water-resistant material, moisture will seep through seams and zippers and saturate your gear if your pack is left unprotected. A pack cover can be anything from a heavy-duty garbage bag, which will keep your pack dry when camping (and protect it from the dew at night), to a specially designed cover made for that purpose. Coated nylon or Gore-Tex covers, when their own seams are properly sealed, fit over your pack, protecting it while you hike. Silk-nylon covers weigh in at about a quarter of coated nylon and Gore-Tex options, while offering comparable protection. They are usually fitted to your pack by elastic or a drawstring.

No matter what kind of pack cover you purchase (and you do need to buy one), you will still want to carry a heavy-duty (BIG) garbage bag to keep your pack covered at night, because pack covers are not designed to protect the straps and back of your pack. A plastic garbage bag is indispensable when you are forced to camp in a downpour but don't have room for your pack in the tent.

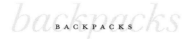

The poncho-style pack covers work under ideal conditions only. The poncho is designed to be a one-piece rain gear, covering both you and your pack at the same time. Not only do ponchos tend to tear easily, but they work only when the wind is not blowing hard. If the wind whips up, so will your poncho; and both you and your pack will soon be soaked. For added insurance, anything you don't want to get wet can be slipped into a plastic bag before being stored in your pack.

OTHER PACK OPTIONS

THE OVERNIGHT OR TWO-DAY PACK

Some hikers can live leanly enough to make long trips with the overnight or two-day type pack. The advantages of the two-day pack are obvious—not only do you carry less weight, but stress on your body is eased. These approximately 2,500- to 3,000-cubic-inch internal-frame packs are definitely not for everyone.

Once again, decide how much you can do without and still enjoy your hike before purchasing a smaller-than-average pack. Two-day/overnight packs range from $80 to $200 for most models. Gregory packs are especially popular.

DAYPACKS

Most daypacks are made in the same teardrop style, so the important thing to look at is how well the pack is made. Inexpensive daypacks can be purchased at any discount store, but if they are poorly padded and have little support, you may regret the purchase within your first mile.

Leather-bottomed packs are the most durable and carry the load better by supporting the weight rather than collapsing beneath it. Make sure the shoulder straps on your daypack are very secure—this is the first place that such packs fall apart. This occurs because you are carrying the weight on your shoulders as opposed to your hips. To prevent ripping, a number of daypacks have extra reinforcement where the shoulder straps connect to the sack. Another feature to look for is padding at the back of the pack. The more reinforced this section, the less likely you'll be poked and prodded by the objects inside the pack.

Features to look for in daypacks include:

- Convenient loading through top or front panel
- Pockets for smaller items (some daypacks feature a special loop to hold keys)
- A waist strap to keep the back from bouncing against your back
- Padded shoulder straps
- Lash points for extra gear

Daypacks are usually less than $100, and most manufacturers feature a variety to choose from.

FANNY PACKS

Another way of keeping things handy is using a fanny pack in conjunction with your backpack. Many hikers use these miniature packs in reverse, snug across their bellies with the strap fastened in the back. Cameras, water, snacks, data books, maps, guides, and anything else to which you need quick access can be carried by this method.

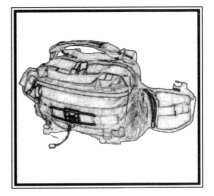

Waist pack
(Mountainsmith Day/Tour)

Fanny packs are useful on day hikes for the same reasons, but they are not as comfortable as daypacks, because they do not distribute the weight as well and often you cannot carry as much as you might like to bring. They can be used along with a daypack or alone (if you have a partner carrying a daypack).

When purchasing a fanny pack, make sure the belt is well padded for comfort and the sack is sturdy enough to carry the load you intend for it. Some fanny packs are designed to carry only very light loads and will sag if heavy objects are placed in them. Also, if the fabric is thin, you may get poked and prodded by the objects inside.

FRAMELESS RUCKSACKS

These approximately 2,500-cubic-inch (and up) packs are gaining a big following. For those backpackers who can travel with the bare minimum and don't need the support and suspension of a framed pack, the rucksack is a great option. This is particularly true for those breaking in to ultralightweight backpacking. Most manufacturers carry frameless packs ranging in price from less than $100 up to $200, or you can sew your own.

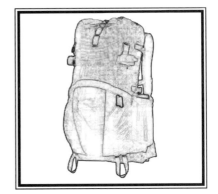

Fastpack rucksack
(GoLite Jam Pack)

HOW MUCH TO CARRY IN YOUR PACK?

There is no easy answer to this question—the amount of weight you carry (within reason) is a matter of personal preference. Usually people new to hiking take far more than they need; as they gain experience, they figure out quickly what is needed on the trail and what they can do without. This is illustrated each spring on the approach trail from Amicalola State Park to the A.T.'s southern terminus on Springer Mountain, where one can sometimes follow jettisoned clothes, food, and equipment as hikers realize they packed too much.

Historically, the advice has been to carry no more than one-third of your body weight. This guideline is probably more appropriate on trails like the Continental Divide Trail and the Pacific Crest Trail, where supply points are few and far between. On most sections of the A.T., though, you won't go more than three to five days before hitting a town, a store, or a highway within easy reach of either. The only exception to this occurs in the Smokies, where it is 70 miles between re-supply points (unless you want to hitch to Gatlinburg) and the "100-Mile Wilderness" in Maine, which, though no longer living up to its moniker, still requires a 62-mile hike before reaching a paved road with access to supplies (at White House Landing).

With this in mind, carrying one-quarter of your weight is reasonable along the A.T. Some hikers swear that you should carry only one-fifth of your body weight, but that can be challenging, especially during winter when the need for warm clothes can add significant weight. It is very important to make sure you carry enough clothing for the worst possible weather (layering will be discussed later) and enough food and water to get you by in case of emergency.

One bit of advice: If you are the organized type, keep a list of what you take each outing. When you return, consult your checklist and consider keeping those items you used over and over again for the next trip and getting rid of those things you used only once or not at all. You can do the same thing if you are thru-hiking: just mail unused or no longer needed stuff back home.

What if you have organized all your gear and food and packed it up, but the pack weighs more than one-quarter of your weight? Unpack and look at everything very carefully. Items like your stove, tent, and sleeping bag are obviously essential, though if money is no object, buying lighter-weight versions of any of these will decrease weight. What about your clothes? You don't have to wear something different every day. And if you must shave, deodorize, shampoo, etc., take along sample-size containers. A radio adds weight too; if you can't do without it, make sure you have the compact "Walkman" type. Flashlights that are "hiker-friendly" can be purchased readily these days; a small flashlight that uses AA batteries will serve you just as well as one that uses C or D batteries, and won't weigh as much. Some thru-hikers go to such extremes as cutting down their toothbrushes, snipping off the edges of topo maps or tearing out sections of guidebooks that won't be used.

These are just a few examples of how much to take. Subsequent chapters also provide suggestions on what to pack. Look objectively at what you've packed: Are you sure you can't live without it?

PACKING YOUR PACK

Once you've bought a pack, where do you put what? You're going to want certain items to be handy. Any system that you come up with will work as long as you know how to get at those necessary items quickly.

Rain gear, for example, will be something that you'll want to be able to lay your hands on immediately. It is not unusual to be caught in a sudden downpour, and if you have to drop your pack and dig through it to get at your raingear, you and all your gear may be soaked by the time you find it.

You will also need a means to carry water so you can get at it without taking off your pack. Some hikers use holsters for their water bottles while others keep their bottles within easy reach in a side pocket on their packs.

Within the pack, it is important to distribute the weight as equally as possible. For example, don't put all your food on one side and all your clothes on the other. Believe it or not, food will be a good third of the weight you are carrying.

Packing the heavier stuff toward the top of your pack will keep the load centered over your hips, particularly in an external-frame pack. On the other hand, don't follow this rule to its furthest possible conclusion, because an overly top-heavy pack is unwieldy.

Sleeping bags are usually secured at the bottom of an external-frame pack, strapped to the frame just below the pack sack. With internal frame packs, the sleeping-bag compartment is usually the bottom third of the pack.

Another suggestion: You will probably want your food more readily available than your clothes and cooking gear, particularly at lunch time. Nothing is more aggravating than digging through your clothes just so you can satisfy a craving for gorp.

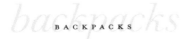

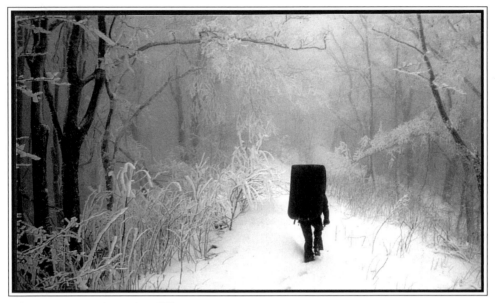

Snow and solitude on the A.T.

LOADING TIPS

- On gentle terrain, pack the heaviest items high and close to the back. Because the pack's center of gravity is about at shoulder level, it will take only a slight bend at the waist while hiking to align the weight over your hips.

- If balance is crucial (climbing, off-trail travel, rough terrain), pack heavy items in the center, close to your back. You may have to lean over more to offset the pack's weight, but balance is better because the pack's top-heaviness is reduced.

- If you are carrying anything sharp in your pack, pad it well. The last thing you want is to be stabbed in the back.

- Women have a lower center of gravity and do well to pack dense items lower and closer to the back.

- Color-coded stuff sacks are a great backpacking tool for organizing gear and food.

- Make sure that all fitting points are properly adjusted to your torso.

- Long items should be lashed to the pack frame.

A Note on Hunting Seasons

If you will be passing through a hunting area (the A.T. passes through numerous Wildlife Management Areas, where hunting seasons usually range from November through February) while hiking along the Appalachian Trail, you might want to take some precautions. Your best bet is to attach something blaze orange to your pack. If you are really concerned, you can always cover your pack with a blaze orange pack cover (sold by the ATC) or even a big orange leaf bag. You could also wear an orange cap. This color is the hunter's signal that something human is approaching, as blaze orange is a color rarely found in the natural world and particularly not moving about two miles per hour through the woods.

For those who are unused to the idea of hunting, the sport is allowed along many parts of the A.T. The regulations for each particular area of the Trail are determined by the land-management agency in that area, of which there are more than 40 along the Trail.

The Trail actually passes through a number of state lands that are managed specifically for hunting, such as the G. Richard Thompson Wildlife Area in northern Virginia or the Pennsylvania State Game Lands.

Check the regulations in each state before hiking. You can find up-to-date information on hunting season posted at the ATC Web site: **www.appalachiantrail.org.**

If your pack is not in your tent with you, leave the pack pockets open at night. Mice, chipmunks, and other rodents have a way of finding packs, particularly at frequently used campsites. If the pockets are open, rodents won't have to chew their way into your pack to search for food.

Chapter Six

Sleeping Bags

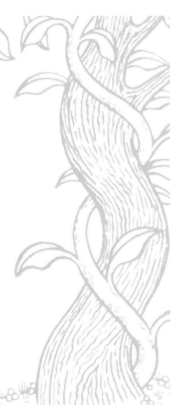

Most people know that a third of their life is spent sleeping. But what many new to backpacking don't know is that there are times when you'll spend even more than a third of your day in a sleeping bag. There come times, particularly on extended backpacking trips, when you can spend as much as 24 to 48 hours stuck in your bag. Inclement weather can send you burrowing into that bag to wait it out. This makes bag choice more important, but fret not—choosing a bag really isn't as daunting as it may seem.

The main traits you should consider when purchasing a bag include comfort rating, type of fill, and weight. The key to sleeping-bag selection is finding the balance point between comfort and practicality that best fits your budget. From there, you can narrow down your options by taking into consideration bag shape and shell material.

IMPORTANT FEATURES
OF SLEEPING BAGS

TEMPERATURE OR COMFORT RATINGS

The first consideration in buying a bag should be how comfortable it will keep you when outdoors. Sleeping-bag manufacturers assign a comfort or temperature rating to their bags to help consumers determine the best bag for their uses. Basically the rating refers to the lowest temperature at which the bag remains comfortable.

Unfortunately, most comfort ratings are overly optimistic and vary widely between manufacturers. The ratings assume you are an average hiker under normal conditions. The problem lies in trying to define who is "average," what conditions are "normal," and what is considered "comfortable." These ratings do not take into account whether or not you are hungry or well fed, hydrated or dehydrated, whether you just hiked 1 mile or 20, or whether it's snowing or the hottest day on record. The ratings also do not reflect the benefits of wearing clothes (you'll be a lot cooler sleeping in the nude and a lot warmer wearing long johns) nor whether you are sleeping in a tent or out in the open (nothing cools you faster than being exposed to bone-chilling wind).

The useful information that comfort ratings provide is the idea of relative warmness. A 10-degree bag will keep you warmer than a 20-degree bag and, when comparing reliable companies, a 20-degree bag from one company will be in the rough ballpark of another's 20-degree bag. This situation should soon be improving. An agreement among 22 European countries will standardize comfort ratings (based on lab tests using a mannequin) for bags sold on the continent. These European ratings should quickly filter into American usage, allowing shoppers to make apple-to-apple comparisons when buying a bag.

Before deciding on a comfort rating, try to determine the range of temperatures in which you will most often be hiking while on the A.T. This can be a challenge, especially for section or thru-hikers, who can cover a wide range of elevation changes (and the ensuing temperature and weather changes) during a trip. It is better to buy a warmer bag (or at least, a bag liner or overbag) than you think you will need than to face a 20-mile day after a cold and sleepless night. If it's too warm to slip into your bag, you can always sleep on top of it! If you intend to do a lot of cold-weather camping, you'll probably want a bag rated between zero and 20 degrees, though for most three-season hiking on the A.T. a 20-degree bag should be adequate. If your hiking will take you through both cold and hot weather, a combination of sleeping bag and bag liner can extend the range in which your bag keeps you warm. Of course, if money is no object, you may prefer to buy several bags with ratings ranging from zero to 45 degrees.

Some people choose to cut down their backpack weight by carrying a blanket (and in one case we know of, a table cloth) instead of a sleeping bag. It is unwise to forfeit your sleeping bag for the sake of weight. Any meteorologist will admit that weather is unpredictable, seemingly changing at whim from hot and muggy to cold and stormy within 24 hours. During our backpacking career, we have had both our coldest and hottest days in Pennsylvania in June. We definitely recommend that you purchase a sleeping bag, even if you only intend to make overnight trips. It's the difference between sleeping warm and shivering wide-awake and could be the difference between life and death.

"You can endure great hardship as long as you can sleep warm."
—Sir Francis Galton, The Art of Travel, 1867

Sleeping-bag Fill

Hard as it might seem to believe, sleeping-bag-fill technology advances almost yearly. Regardless, there are six main categories into which these stuffers have been delegated: down, the old synthetics, the new or short staple synthetics, the continuous-filament synthetics, pile or fleece, and proprietary synthetics. Keep in mind that the pri-

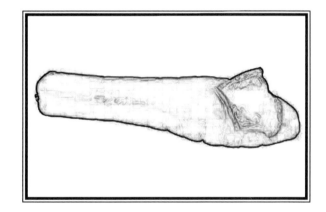

Down bag (GoLite Feather Bag)

mary concern that should influence your decision when choosing a fill is what happens to that fill when it gets wet, though weight and packability are also important concerns. Once again, your choice will be a question of preference.

Down: Down has long been lauded and is still number one when it comes to providing maximum warmth and comfort for minimum weight and bulk. Down

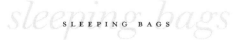

sleeping bags breathe better than polyester fiber bags and are less stifling in warmer temperatures than their synthetic counterparts. But when a down bag gets wet, it loses almost all of its ability to warm and gains much more in weight than synthetic bags. Down bags also mat and clump worse than synthetic bags. Down bags are notoriously bad for hay-fever sufferers. If you're allergic to feather pillows, you'll be allergic to down bags.

Both goose down and duck down are used as fillings, with the difference discernible only under a microscope. But goose down is generally considered structurally superior. The fill power or loft of down is measured in cubic inches and simply represents the number of cubic inches 1 ounce of down will expand to in a 24-hour period. For example, 600 cubic inches is considered to be a superior loft, 500 to 550 is very good, and so on. That infamous "do not remove" tag will inform you of the bag's loft. By the way, for you, ultralight hikers, the consumer is allowed to remove the tag once the product has been purchased.

"OLD SYNTHETICS": Quallofil and Hollofil/Hollofil II. You can find these synthetic fills in the budget bags these days although just a few years ago they were considered state-of-the-art. While they will keep you warm when they get wet, these fillings are a lot heavier and bulkier than the newer synthetics.

Quallofil fibers are hollow, and feature four microscopic tubes that allow for good insulating ability and increase fiber surface area. This polyester filling, which is as soft as down, is nonallergenic and retains most of its loft when wet so that it doesn't become thin and hard or lose its warmth.

A type of polyester, Hollofil fibers are about two inches long and must be sewn to a backing to prevent clumping; this leads to cold spots in a sleeping bag. Similar to Quallofil, Hollofil has a single hole in the fiber; but it allows for more "air" per ounce and thus provides more insulation. The added insulation is gained at a price because the backing materials used for the filling add weight. Like other polyester fills, Hollofil loses only about a tenth of its warmth when wet. The newer Hollofil II has silicone added to make the fibers easier to compress and the bag, therefore, easier to push into a stuff sack.

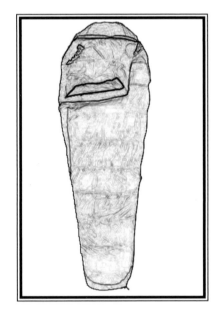

Synthetic bag
(The North Face Cat's Meow)

NEW OR SHORT STAPLE SYNTHETICS: Lite Loft, Micro-loft, Primaloft, Primaloft 2, Thermolite Extra, Thermolite Extreme. These fills come pretty close to matching down's warmth and softness. They are also a good deal lighter and more packable than down. But, unlike down, heavy-duty use reduces their loft.

Thinsulate Lite Loft by 3M is the warmest synthetic insulation available for its weight. Its microfine polyester/olefin fibers make it lightweight even when wet and easily compressible. Microloft is made by Du Pont and boasts the smallest of the microfibers. These tiny fibers enable Microloft to trap more heat and remain soft and supple. The Primalofts mimic the structure of goose down with tiny fibers interspersed with stiffer fibers. Unlike down, Primaloft is water repellent and retains its warmth when wet.

CONTINUOUS-FILAMENT SYNTHETICS: Polarguard, Polarguard HV, Polarguard 3D, and Polarguard Delta. More durable than the short staple synthetics, these fibers, which are long and interwoven, don't become matted, which eliminates the need for a backing to prevent cold spots. Polarguard HV also retains its loft—thus its warmth when wet. The new Polarguard Delta and Polarguard 3D perform best, though they tend to be bulkier and heavier than the short-staple synthetics.

PILE OR FLEECE: Pile works great for a jacket, so why not a sleeping bag? The bulky material tends to be used in inexpensive bags. Though fairly lightweight, they are really only used in a few warm-weather sleeping bags and are not a good three-season option. Some overbags and bag liners use fleece to help boost your sleeping bag's rating for colder weather.

PROPRIETARY SYNTHETICS: These are synthetic fills produced by the manufacturers of some sleeping bags to fill their own bags. Quality varies according to manufacturer. You will want to check the Internet for online ratings of these by other hikers before making a purchase.

According to tests conducted by Recreational Equipment Incorporated (REI), "a synthetic bag will lose about 10 percent of its warmth while gaining about 60 percent in weight" when the sleeping bag gets wet. Conversely, they report that a water-soaked, down-filled bag "will lose over 90 percent of its warmth, gain 128 percent in weight, and take more than a day to dry."

What this means is that your ability to keep a down bag dry is a major factor when deciding to purchase a bag. All six fills have strong proponents. When purchasing a bag, decide how much trouble you want to go through to keep your bag dry. Stuffing your sleeping bag into a plastic garbage bag before putting it in a stuff sack will keep it dryer. And if you will be fording a stream or are expecting hard rains, put the stuff sack into another bag for extra protection.

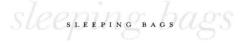

WEIGHT

In conjunction with comfort rating and fill, weight is the third element in considering which bag to buy. Weight is related to the comfort and fill rating. Usually, the lower the comfort rating, the more the bag weighs. However, within a given comfort rating, bags will vary quite significantly given different fills. Generally, the lightest bag that gives you the greatest warmth for your comfort needs is best. Unfortunately, the lighter the bag, the more it's going to cost. As a rule, do not buy a bag that weighs more than five pounds. For A.T. backpackers, a bag in the two- to four-pound range is probably the best bet for cost-efficiency and warmth.

Keep in mind that it is likely that the bag you buy will eventually get wet, and that its weight will increase as a result.

OTHER BAG CONSIDERATIONS

SHAPE

Sleeping bags come in three basic shapes: mummy, rectangular, and semirectangular. Most backpackers choose the mummy-shaped bag because it offers the most warmth and space for the least weight. Most bags offer what is called a draft tube behind the zipper to prevent air from leaking into the bag. If you intend to use your bag in windy or even cool weather be sure that the bag you choose has a draft tube.

MUMMY: The name describes the shape. Formed to the contours of your body, the mummy has the least amount of air to warm and takes less material to make (and, therefore, to stuff). This saves on weight as well. The mummy's "head" is designed to draw down over and around your own on cold nights, limiting your body's heat loss. Most mummy bags also feature a "boxed" foot section, which keeps the insulation in place over your feet so that they stay warmer. But like everything, the mummy has its drawbacks. There is absolutely no room to turn around in it. You either toss and turn the entire bag or sleep in one position through the night. Also, the short zippers hamper ventilation.

RECTANGULAR: This is the roomiest and the heaviest of sleeping bags. Three sides of the bag are zippered, allowing you to ventilate to the point of making the bag a blanket. Room and ventilation become the bag's drawbacks on cold nights because there is more air to heat and no hood to prevent heat from escaping through your head.

SEMIRECTANGULAR: This bag has the taper of a mummy bag without the hood. The design saves some on weight, provides good ventilation because it, too, is zippered on three sides, and has a bit less air to heat up. Like the rectangular bag, there is no hood for cold nights. It is a good choice for large-framed hikers who don't mind carrying the few extra ounces.

When purchasing a sleeping bag, make sure it fits. A bag that is too narrow or too short will affect the quality of your sleep. Because a mummy bag follows the contours of your body, make sure that it is not too tight in the shoulders and around your head. If you are planning extended backpacking and/or cold-weather trips, you may want to buy a bag with extra room at the feet. The extra room will accommodate water bottles, boots, socks, or any other things you may want to keep from freezing.

SHELLS

Another important consideration when buying a bag is the shell or outer covering. Although there are numerous materials to choose from, you will want to consider only shells made from DryLoft, Epic, Microfiber, Pertex Endurance, ripstop, and taffeta.

DryLoft is made by W. L. Gore and is a highly breathable and water-resistant fabric. DryLoft is very similar to Gore-Tex and will hold at bay wind, condensation, and light rain. In a sleeping bag with a DryLoft shell, you can sleep under the stars or in a snow cave without having to worry about waking up cold and wet.

Epic by Nextec encloses polyester microfibers in a very thin silicon-based polymer film. A durable, breathable barrier is then created between the fiber bundles. The soft fabric allows body vapor to escape, keeping you drier.

Microfiber is a tightly woven nylon or polyester fabric that is usually more supple and lighter than DryLoft. It is, on the other hand, less resistant to water than both DryLoft and Gore-Tex. But it does repel wind and breathe well.

Pertex Endurance faired well in a 2004 *Backpacker* magazine test claiming that this material "raises the bar for repelling moisture." The only negative is that many bags made with the fabric are not seam-sealed and not as water repellent as they would otherwise be.

Ripstop nylon and polyester feature heavier threads interwoven in the fabric every quarter inch or so in a checkerboard or diamond pattern to prevent rips from running down the bag. It also forms a web of reinforcement to reduce stress. Strong for its weight, ripstop nylon is also wind resistant. On the other hand, it does not repel water and therefore gets wet easily—although it dries quickly.

Taffeta is a flat-weave fabric that is softer than ripstop but isn't as strong or as resistant to wind. It, too, gets wet easily. Nylon taffeta is often used as an inner lining.

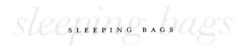

As with sleeping-bag fillings, some manufacturers make their own proprietary shell materials, which are hard to assess. Once again, checking online ratings at a site like **www.epinions.com** can help separate the reality from the manufacturer's potentially hyped advertising.

MATED BAGS

For couples interested in hiking, some sleeping bags may be zipped together. Many sleeping bag manufacturers offer bags with right and left zippers. If you intend to buy mateable bags, you may want to consider one lightweight (approximately 40-degree) and one heavier (about 20-degree) bag. That way, if it's warm, you can use the cooler bag on top—and vice versa.

ADDED FEATURES

Some extra features you might want to keep in mind when purchasing a sleeping bag include:

OPTIONAL FABRICS: Some manufacturers will allow you to pick which shell fabric you want on the bag.

BRUSHED INNER LINING: This fleecy lining feels soft and cozy on cold nights. On muggy nights, this lining can wick away the perspiration from your body but some people claim the lining holds in too much heat.

INSULATED DRAFT COLLAR: This is a puffy yoke or collar that can be cinched closely around your neck (usually with a drawstring) to keep the warm air in the bag and the cold drafts out of it. A draft collar makes a huge difference in how warm you stay on a cold night.

HOOD: As most people know, most of your body's heat is lost through the head. That's what makes wearing a hat so important in cold weather and, similarly, what makes having a hood on your sleeping bag so important in frigid conditions. Look for a hood with a contoured cut that is snug but not too tight and that features plenty of insulation. Some hoods use elastic to snug the hood, others feature a drawstring.

POCKET: Some sleeping bags feature a zippered pocket at chest level to provide you with handy storage of things you might want to keep close by, such as contact lenses, a flashlight or headlamp, and lip balm. This works well for those who can maintain a single position throughout the night.

STORAGE BAG: This is a big, breathable cotton bag designed to prolong the life of your bag when you are not using it. If you cram your bag into its stuff sack and forget about it for a few months, it will lose its loft.

ZIPPER OPTIONS: This essentially means that you can choose whether or not you want a right-handed zipper or a left-handed zipper or whether or not the zipper can be mated with another sleeping bag.

INSULATED ZIPPER DRAFT TUBE: This is basically a draft collar for your zipper and is a wonderful option. The tube should hang from the top of the zipper so that it stays in place over the teeth.

WOMAN'S MODELS: Some sleeping bags are designed with a woman's needs specifically in mind, particularly some models from Sierra Designs. What does that mean? Usually these bags feature extra width at the hips and less at the shoulders, more insulation in the foot box, and less overall length.

CARING FOR YOUR BAG

Synthetic sleeping bags can be washed by hand or in a commercial washer with warm or cold water. They should be cleaned with a mild soap such as Ivory, and, if not air dried, they should be dried at a low setting in your dryer. When air-drying any bag, make sure it is well supported. Never hang it by one end because the weight of the wet filling may tear out the inner construction and ruin the bag. Supporting the bag on a slanted board is a good option. Don't wash your sleeping bag after every trip. That stresses the fabric. Rather, wash it only when it is really dirty.

Down sleeping bags should be hand washed. If washed in a machine, your bag could lose its loft because the detergent breaks down the natural oils of the goose down. Down bags should not be dried in a household dryer; rather, they should be drip dried for several days. The bag can then be placed in a commercial dryer on low heat to fluff it. Throwing in a clean pair of tennis shoes will break up matted down.

Sleeping bags should not be stored in the tiny stuff sacks that they are normally carried in on a hike. A big, loose bag is the best container for keeping your bag in good condition when you're not on the trail. Stuffing your bag into a small sack every day while hiking is all right because you're taking your bag out almost every night. But if you store it that way at home, the filling becomes packed together and it is hard to restore its loft. Never roll your bag up neatly because this compresses the insulation. Stuffing the bag into its sack assures you of a different pattern of compression each day, which is better on the loft.

Another way to increase the life of your bag is to wash up each night before crawling into it. The dirt and oil on your clothes and body will find its way into your bag's fill and inhibit its ability to insulate. If you can't wash up, change into clean clothes.

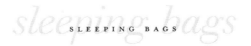

SLEEPING-BAG ACCESSORIES

BAG LINERS

Purchasing a bag liner is a good way to warm up your bag without adding much cost or weight. There are three types of bag liners: overbags, vapor barriers, and plain inner liners.

OVERBAGS: An overbag slides over your sleeping bag and has a fill that increases the warmth of your bag by as much as 20 degrees. They cost approximately $50 to $100 and weigh about two to three pounds—kind of bulky for extensive backpacking but not too bad for short, cold-weather trips.

VAPOR BARRIERS: These liners are inserted inside your sleeping bag and can raise its temperature by as much as 15 degrees. Basically, with the vapor barrier, you're sticking yourself inside a plastic bag. They are constructed out of coated nylon or other materials and weigh only five to six ounces. Also, they cost much less than the overbags—approximately $20 to $30. The drawback to the vapor barrier is comfort; they make you sweat and use your own warmth to keep you warm. Vapor liners are recommended for temperatures well below freezing.

PLAIN INNER LINERS: You can also purchase simple bag liners made of flannel, cotton, breathable nylon, synthetics, and down, costing anywhere from $5 to $100 and weighing three ounces to two pounds. The degree to which they warm your bag varies and should be clarified by the salesperson before you decide to purchase such a liner.

SLEEPING PADS

Sleeping pads are a necessity. If you don't sleep on a pad, you lose your heat to the ground. Although the padding is minimal, they are more comfortable than the hard earth. Fortunately, as with all things backpacking-gear related, there are plenty of pads to choose from, and you are sure to find one that meets your needs.

CLOSED-CELL FOAM: This type of pad features tiny plastic bubbles squeezed together in a honeycomb-style. These are both inexpensive and lightweight and they shed water to boot. Closed-cell foam is also pretty durable. Its drawback? It needs to be relatively thick to block out those roots and rocks and, of course, the thicker the pad, the bulkier.

OPEN-CELL FOAM: This is the opposite of the closed-cell pad. Think egg-crate mattress, and you get the general idea. This type of pad always reminds me of the inside of an egg carton and is frequently used in hospitals for bed-ridden patients. This pad offers excellent comfort and contours, is inexpensive, and packs down small. Unless it has a waterproof coating though, it becomes a sponge in the vicinity of water.

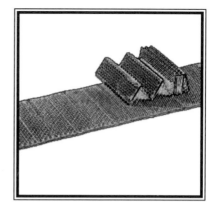

Sleeping pad
(Therm-a-Rest Z-Lite)

SELF-INFLATING PAD: Who hasn't heard the one about the hiker who was like a Therm-A-Rest? That's right! Self-inflating! This is an open-cell foam pad encased in a watertight, airtight cover. It is fitted with a valve to allow you to inflate it. This is achieved by unscrewing the valve, unrolling the pad, and waiting while the foam rebounds, drawing in air, and returns it to its original shape. This pad provides the best comfort available. But, of course, it has its drawbacks, too. It is expensive, on the heavy side, and susceptible to puncture.

OTHER MATERIALS: Other pad options include those filled with heat reflective materials and those filled with down.

After deciding on which type of pad you want to purchase, you might also want to look into the different features available in pads these days. One of the most popular pad features are pads that convert to chairs. These pads have buckles and straps that allow you to turn your sleeping pad into a camp chair. You can also buy a conversion kit that will turn any pad into a chair.

Some pads come with what are known as *integral compression* or roll straps. These make shrinking and packing your pad a bit easier. The straps also give you more options when it comes to attaching the pad on the outside of your pack.

Pads with *multiple chambers* allow you to over-inflate one section without creating an annoying bubble elsewhere. Another bonus is that should the pad puncture, only one chamber will deflate rather than the entire pad. The seams between pads affect the insulation on these pads, though. Cold air can creep through at these junctures.

Some closed-cell pads feature a *molded surface* that is dimpled or ridged. They are preferable to the flat models due to less slippage, better cushioning, and less weight.

A new gimmick to save on weight and bulk is the *mummy-shaped* pad. The main drawback is that you need to be one of those people who sleeps soundly and doesn't move around a lot in your sleep otherwise you might find your feet slipping off the tapered bottom section.

Another kind of cool feature of pads is the *no-slip surface*. A brushed or sticky surface on your sleeping pad helps your sleeping bag maintain the traction it needs to stay on your pad, especially on uneven campsites.

Some pads come with an *attached pillow*, but these tend to be bulky and most hikers can do with a rolled-up jacket or sweater beneath their head.

Two other features you might want to look for are the *repair kit* and *stuff sack*. The former is particularly important because a few patches and fix-it glue might make the difference between a good night's sleep and waking up on the wrong side of the sleeping bag. A stuff sack is just added insurance against trail grime and possible puncture if you have a self-inflating pad.

When it comes to determining the thickness, weight, and length of your pad, your own preferences are the best judge. You know how much padding you need and how much weight you can carry. Your height, too, will affect how long your pad needs to be.

Pillows

Some people cannot sleep without a pillow. Whenever I hike, I use my pile jacket as a pillow. I carry it anyway so there's not the added bulk of a camping pillow. I consider camp pillows needless weight even on short backpacking trips, but for those of you who wish to carry the extra half-pound, you have the choice of a small (10–12 by 16–20 inches) synthetic stuffed pillow or an inflatable pillow. Relatively inexpensive, backpacking pillows are a matter of preference.

Pack your sleeping bag into a garbage bag before loading it into its stuff sack. This will keep the day's rain from ruining a good night's sleep. This is critical with down sleeping bags, which loose their ability to insulate when wet. If you will be fording a stream or are expecting hard rains, put the stuff sack into another bag to doubly protect your sleeping bag.

How Can You Sleep More Peacefully?

Try these time-tested tips:

- Make sure your bag fits you. If the bag is too tight then the insulation will compress and will be unable to do its job. And, if it is too loose, you will expend extra energy trying to heat up the additional space, draining your energy reserves before dawn breaks. If possible, wear whatever you intend to sleep in when trying out bags. And don't even think about sleeping naked when it is cold!

- Don't forget to cinch the draft collar and your hood (if you have them). This will keep you much warmer.

- Keep your bag from getting wet at all costs. Store it in a waterproof stuff sack and carry extra garbage bags to store the stuff sack in on wet days. And never, ever, climb into a sleeping bag wet. As a matter of fact, if you're facing hypothermia, it is better to crawl into your bag naked than into your bag with wet clothes on. Make sure you change into dry clothes as soon as possible.

- If it is possible that you will get cold during the night, keep some extra clothes nearby along with a hat (if you are not already wearing one) to slip on when you start feeling the chill through your sleeping bag.

- Make yourself an old-fashioned foot warmer with a Nalgene or other leak-proof bottle filled with warm or hot water.

- Make sure you eat well before heading off to dreamland. This helps keep your energy level high enough to ward off the chill.

- Make sure you empty your bladder before you crawl into your bag. Believe it or not, it takes energy to keep that liquid warm, and you won't waste the stored heat in your bag by getting out of your bag to pee.

- If it looks to be a cold night, try at least 20 jumping jacks (or other calisthenics) before heading into the sack. If you get cold during the night, crawl out of your bag and do some more.

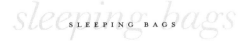

Chapter Seven

Footgear

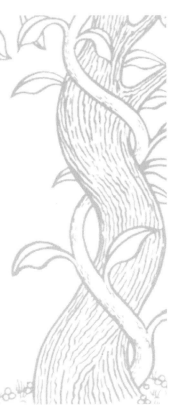

Within the past generation, hiking boots have come of age. Twenty or so years ago, boots were all leather, heavy as all get out, and that was it. Today, you have proponents of lightweight, mediumweight, and heavyweight boots, those who swear by their cross trainers or jogging shoes, and those who will wear nothing but sport sandals. What you choose to wear is up to you. There are certainly times when it is just as easy to maneuver a trail in cross trainers as in Vasques. And when it comes to stream crossings, there has been many an occasion when we have slipped on Tevas to both protect our feet and keep our boots from getting wet. Almost every hiker can tell you a boot story—from dissolving uppers and disappearing soles to swamp rot and ulcerous blisters. The shoes you choose can protect or destroy your feet. And since backpacking usually involves being on your feet all day, boots that fit comfortably will be your most important gear acquisition.

SELECTING YOUR
HIKING SHOES

B efore you go out and buy just any old boot, you need to decide what type of hiking you plan on doing. Do you plan to go on the occasional weekend trip, or do you intend to be on the trail weeks at a time. Your selection of boots will also depend on where and when you want to hike. Hiking strictly on smooth, established trails requires a different boot than hiking off-trail through a rocky landscape. Generally, the longer you will be out and the heavier the pack, the heavier the boot you need.

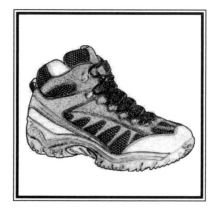

*Lightweight boot
(Merrell Mesa Ventilator)*

Traditionally boots have been referred to as light-, medium-, or heavyweight. *Lightweight* boots weigh less than 2.5 pounds per pair, rarely require an extended breaking-in period, are more flexible, and have shallower lug outsoles. Usually made of fabric, they cost between $60 and $100. Lightweight boots are the best choice for day trips and light hiking on easy terrain. One of the most popular choices for A.T. hiking, *mediumweight* boots weigh between 2.5 and 4 pounds and are either half-fabric/half-leather or all-leather. Wider outsoles and heavy-duty midsoles, combined with a half-length to three-quarters-length steel shank, help to protect feet from bruising stones. They usually cost between $100 and $170. Rock scrambling and rougher terrain call for mediumweight boots. *Heavyweight* boots usually weigh 4 pounds or more and cost over $200. They are made of thicker, stiffer leather than mediumweights. They have close-trimmed soles and a half- to full-length steel shank in the sole. These boots are designed for technically demanding hiking, particularly where snow and ice will be encountered.

However, keep in mind that buying a particular boot does not predispose you to one particular activity. Certainly buying a heavyweight boot to use only on

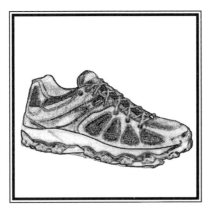

Cross trainers (Dunham Waffle Stomper Nimble)

occasional weekends is fine, and if you feel comfortable with lightweight boots on extended hikes, that's your choice.

Though boots are still referred to by weight, manufacturers and retailers have started to categorize footwear by the activity for which they are appropriate. Here's how they breakdown:

RUNNING SHOES: You do not have to wear boots to backpack. Well-built running shoes will suffice on the entire A.T. The move toward ultralightweight backpacking has particularly spurred on the move away from boots. When carrying a pack of less than 35 pounds, the need for beefed up shoes diminishes. Ankle support is helpful, but not essential for everyone. As with any type of footwear, try out running shoes on a shorter shakedown hike before committing to them for the long haul.

TRAIL OR CROSS-TRAIL: Basic trail boots combine fabric and leather or split-leather construction, with uppers that come below the ankle, though occasionally you'll see some that are ankle high. They also usually have multiple seams, which allows for more moisture to enter your boots and thus dampen your socks. If the boot doesn't have a waterproof/breathable liner, you'll need to purchase some Gore-Tex socks or apply some waterproofing as well as carry along some gaiters for "just in case." Lightweight boots have stiffer soles, more stability, and better traction than running or walking shoes, but they can be unstable on slippery or rocky terrain.

TECHNICAL SCRAMBLING, ALL TERRAIN, OR APPROACH: These can be both lightweight and mediumweight boots designed for basic boulder scrambling and light trail use. They are usually below-ankle and ankle-high boots that hug the foot closely. They have sticky rubber soles for traction as well as anti-abrasion toe rands. They provide enough support to carry a light backpack on well-maintained trails, but if you're planning on doing major miles with a heavy pack, you'll want a more substantial boot.

ROUGH TRAIL, TREKKING, HIKING, OR TRAIL SPORT: These are mediumweight boots made from a leather/fabric combination or thin splits of grain leather. They are perfect for easy, short backpacking trips when you are not carrying a too-heavy pack. Some of these boots have waterproof/breathable liners, and others are porous and well ventilated for desert hiking. They tend to have tapered plastic midsoles or half-length shanks, which provide enough sole rigidity to protect your feet on rocky trails but still allow good flex at the balls of the feet.

OFF TRAIL, BACKPACKING, OR BACK-COUNTRY: These are heavyweight boots designed for bushwhacking across unknown terrain (unknown to you, at least). They are made with full-grain leather, above-the-ankle support, and rigid sole stability. They are best for long backpacking trips because they offer plenty of

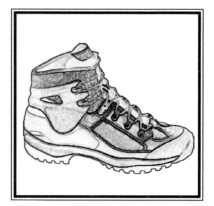

Midweight boot
(Lowa Vertex GTX)

protection beneath heavy loads, yet provide enough flex at the balls of your feet to be comfortable. If you put enough miles on these boots, they will eventually become very supple, but it can take a long time for the sole and the heel-cup to soften. Off-trail boots also offer excellent waterproofing and durability because they have a minimum number of seams. With new boot technology, many of these formerly "heavyweight" boots are now a lot lighter. Some models have a lip on the welt of the sole to handle step-in crampons or the new snowshoe bindings if you intend to do some winter hiking along the northern A.T.

MOUNTAINEERING OR ALPINE: Tough, rugged, and heavy, these are the boots that have that NASA look. They are made for high, cold, and mountainous terrain. Made of plastic or thick, full-grain leather uppers, these boots rise well above the ankle and have full-length shanks or stiff nylon midsoles, making them too rigid for normal backpacking. Unless you are going to hike through ice and snow fields, don't bother with these boots.

Note: Regardless of weight or style, boots made with waterproof Gore-Tex (look for the GTX) often cost $30 or $40 more.

BOOT CONSTRUCTION

UPPERS

There are numerous types of uppers, or the portion of the boot above the sole: full-grain leather, split-grain leather (inner hide split off the waterproof and supportive outside), Nubuk leather (sanded full-grain leather), synthetic fabrics (often used in combination with leather), Gore-Tex, other proprietary water-proof/breathable membranes (which are added inside the leather or fabric upper), and plastic. Because of its support, breathability, comfort, protectiveness, and ability to be waterproofed, leather is most often used when constructing uppers. The highest-quality boots feature an all-leather upper because there is less stitching for water to leak through and fewer seams to burst. Multiple-piece leather uppers are your next best option, because they cost less than all-leathers and can be waterproofed.

Fabric/leather uppers reinforce canvas or nylon with pieces of leather to help the boots resist abrasion and to increase support. For boots that combine fabric and leather, you will want to use a silicon-based waterproofing treatment, such as Nikwax Aqueous.

Uppers made of plastic are used only in heavyweight mountaineering boots. Although light, warm, strong, and waterproof, plastic uppers are too rigid for most terrains.

Uppers also include cuffs or scree collars that are stitched to the ankle top of most boots to provide some protection against the inevitable invasion of pebbles and twigs. Internal cuffs are better than external because they last longer.

The tongue of the boot should be gussetted for the best protection against moisture and debris. The gusset is a thin piece of leather or other material sewn between the boot upper and tongue. The best protection is found in a bellows tongue, which has a full-length gusset that covers the entire tongue opening. Overlapping tongues also provide a nearly watertight closure. Well-padded tongues are more comfortable, offering some protection against tightly laced boots.

The protective piece of leather sewn over the back seam of most boots is called the backstay. Because it is next to impossible to replace, look for a backstay that is narrow. It will be less vulnerable to abrasion.

Toe and heel counters are also part of a well-made upper. These are stiffeners built into the toe and heel areas to provide some protection against rocks and roots.

SOLES

The outsole, midsole, and steel shank make up the sole of the boot. The outsole, often a Vibram product, usually has either shallow or deep lugs to provide traction. Good traction is particularly important if you intend to do some rock scrambling or if you will be gaining and losing a lot of elevation while carrying a heavy pack. While shallow lugs are designed for easy-to-moderate terrain and are usually paired with lightweight boots, deeper lugs can be found on mediumweight and heavyweight boots and provide the traction needed for most backpacking trips.

Between the outsole and insole of the boot is the midsole. The thickness of the midsole varies with the boot but is designed to provide extra protection, extra support, and cushioning between your foot and the ground. Even lightweight boots feature a midsole, often of EVA or polyurethane, for added comfort.

Most boots have a steel (or plastic or nylon) shank that ensures that the sole of your boot flexes at the ball of your foot. Except for plastic boots, which have an inherently rigid sole, shanks range in length from a quarter- to full-length. The lightweight boots usually require only up to a half-length shank, while the mediumweight to heavyweight boots need at least a half- to full-length shank for optimum rigidity.

Some boots have a rockered (curved) sole for a more natural stride, minimal heel slippage, and rubber bands along the welt for durability and waterproofing. I can't imagine that you would need these types of boots for hiking along the A.T., even in Maine!

LEATHER

There are several different methods used to cure and tan the leather that makes up the hundreds of boots designed for hiking, backpacking, and mountaineering. Placing hides in a rotating drum containing a solution of chromium sulfate is called chrome tanning, and all leather undergoes this first process. Some leathers then undergo a vegetable process that involves tanning with plant derivatives. This step gives the leather extra body and solidity. Some leathers are put through a step called fatliquoring in which the leather is cured with either oils to make it softer, or waxes to make it firmer.

Hide straight off the cow is too thick for even the heaviest of boots. All leather is split into sheets of varying thickness. Full-grain leather, the outside layer of the hide, is the highest-quality leather—resistant to abrasion, the most waterproof, and the stiffest. All other layers are called "splits." Quality of splits varies but only the layer beneath the full-grain can be used in boots, and it must be specially treated to make it resistant to water.

Most manufacturers use full-grain leather in their uppers. Because of the battering hiking boots receive, many manufacturers will turn the full-grain leather inside out before stitching it to the sole. This way, the water-resistant side faces inward and is less likely to receive nicks and scratches from rocks and roots, which will allow water to seep into your boot. How can you tell which way the full-grain is facing? The outside of the boot will be smooth if the top layer is out, rough if the top layer is facing in. Boots designed for easy hiking often have the top layer facing out.

THE WELT

The importance of the welt (or how the upper is fastened to the sole) never occurred to me until Frank lost the soles of his New Balance Cascades outside of Elk Park, North Carolina. Hiking 60 miles to the next town with his soles duct-taped to his uppers was pure torture, but what if a friendly hiker hadn't had the tape? A bare-footed jaunt to the next road carrying a 40-pound pack was unthinkable. . . so carry duct tape (probably one of the better modern inventions along with WD-40—just ask MacGyver) and check out the welt on the boots you plan to hike in. The welt is usually accomplished with stitching and/or cement and affects both the strength and flexibility of the boot.

The Goodyear welt is accomplished with two rows of stitching. A horizontal stitch joins the upper to both the insole and a strip of leather. This strip of leather is then vertically stitched to the soles. This welt is very flexible and is often used in lightweight hiking boots. Both the outer and midsole can be replaced on boots using this welt.

The Norwegian welt also uses two rows of stitching—a horizontal stitch to join the upper and lining to the insole, and a vertical stitch to attach the upper to the midsole. While not as flexible as the Goodyear welt, the Norwegian welt is much stronger and is often used in mediumweight and heavyweight boots. Outer and midsoles can also be replaced on this boot.

Another type of welt is called the "inside fastened," the "Littleway," or the "McKay." This welt is achieved by rolling the upper between the insole and midsole and then stitching all three together from the inside. This is both a flexible and durable welt method and is often used on lightweight hiking boots. Like the other methods, both the outer and midsoles can be replaced.

Because they are not intended for heavy use, lightweight boots often have cement-welted soles. A narrow outsole is required, which can be a drawback. Advances in technology have produced strong adhesives, but boots with soles that are attached with an epoxy take a bit of extra care.

Don't dry them out too close to a heat source because the epoxy could melt, and a few miles down the trail the sole could separate from the upper.

FITTING YOUR BOOTS

Select your boot carefully. Backpacking is an activity that often involves spending the entire day on your feet as well as putting an extraordinary amount of weight on them. The strongest welt, toughest leather, and supertraction soles

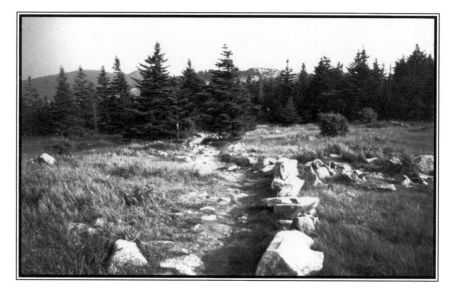

Rocky terrain of southwest Virginia

will mean little if every step is agonizing because of improper fit. You may be proud of your small, shapely feet, but buying a boot because it enhances your appearance is foolish and may amount to a face lined with anguish by day's end.

Boot sizing is notorious for its inconsistency. You might normally wear a size 6 in tennis shoes but a 5 or a 7 in a boot. Make sure that the boots are not only long enough for you but wide enough as well. A number of boots come in several widths: find the one that's right for you.

The most important thing when purchasing a boot is whether or not it is comfortable. When trying on the boot, wear hiking socks. A boot might feel comfy over a thin cotton crew, but slip it on over a thick polypropylene sock and suddenly your foot feels like a sardine. Also, if you intend to wear insoles, which give you extra cushioning and arch support, bring them along when you are trying on boots, because insoles also affect the way a boot fits.

How do you know if the fit is big enough but not too big? Is there a thumb's width between your toes and the tip of your boot? Can you wiggle your toes for good circulation? Take all the time you need to get a good fit.

While my first pair of boots didn't give me blisters, they were too short. On the downhill, my feet slid forward into the toe of the boot, resulting in painfully numb toes that throbbed all night long. Not even aspirin could dim that pain. Long-distance hikers often lose toenails. A boot that is long enough will help alleviate that problem. On the other hand, make sure your heel doesn't slip. This could lead to blisters. The heel should be snug but it shouldn't pinch you.

Lace your boots up securely. Is there any part of the boot that is uncomfortable? Pressure should be even all over your foot, which contains more than 26 bones. Tell the salesperson what you feel. Is there unusual pressure at the instep? Let him or her know. They'll probably suggest a boot that will suit you better.

Finally, don't be surprised if you can't find a perfect fit. With more than 132 potential foot shapes, no manufacturer can fit everyone. Once you've found the next-best thing to perfect, the boot can probably be altered with orthotics and broken in to fit.

WATERPROOFING

If your boots have any leather in their construction, they need waterproofing. Sno-Seal, and the newer Aquaseal, are two popular brands of sealant although there are a number of others. Devoutly follow directions for the waterproofer you purchase. Dry feet make all the difference in the world!

Unfortunately, sealing your boots is not a one-time deal. It must be done periodically; and the more you use your boots, the more often you must seal them. For hikes of more than a week or two, you may want to carry sealant along with you. Or send some ahead if you plan to have mail drops.

Taking care of your boots will ensure a longer lifespan (for your boots, that is). After every backpacking trip, brush off dirt and debris before storing. If your boots are wet, try stuffing them with newspaper to soak up the inside moisture and let them dry in a cool, dry place. Don't try to dry them quickly by setting them near a heater, oven, or open flame. It could mean the death of your boots. Once they are dry, reseal them with waterproofer. Seams and welts and the leather used in lightweight boots require a special sealant. All boot sealants can be purchased in outdoors stores.

LACES AND LACING

While leather laces used to be popular, their tendency to stretch when wet has been their demise. Nylon has replaced them as the standard lace for hiking boots. The durable, soft-woven, unwaxed nylon laces also hold knots best.

Hiking boots usually feature three different methods of closure—grommets, D rings, and hooks. Lacing using only grommets is probably the sturdiest; grommets usually last well past the lifetime of the boot. The only problem with an all-grommet boot is that it can be difficult to lace, particularly when your hands are blocks of ice. Many boots have grommets in the lower half of the boot and hooks at the top.

My boots have D rings on the lower half and hooks above. They are very easy to lace, even with numb fingers (it's the knot I have trouble with when I can't even feel the laces).

There are a few tips to keep in mind when lacing your boots. If the upper knot of your boot rubs against your shin, lace your boots to the top then back down a few notches, and tie the knot midway down your boot to prevent a painful bruise. Another advantage of this method is that it keeps the knot from loosening under the pressure of your constantly bending ankle.

If your toes are feeling cramped, try loosening up the lower laces a bit, tie a knot, and continue lacing the boot tightly. This could backfire on the downhill if the loose laces cause your toes to slide painfully into the front of your boot. In this case, you might want to try the opposite approach.

EXTRA SHOES

Should you carry an extra pair of shoes with you when you hike? Well, that all depends on the distance you're hiking. For day trips, you won't need an extra pair of shoes. Weekenders and section hikers, and especially long-distance hikers, should carry a pair of camp shoes to lessen their impact around camp. Lightweight, soft-soled shoes cause less compaction of the soil and trampling of vegetation, especially if you are intending to camp in pristine areas.

If you are going to be out for more than a few days, you need to seriously consider additional footwear. We've seen all kinds carried: tennis shoes, espadrilles, flip-flops, clogs, aqua socks, sandals.

There are a number of reasons to carry additional footwear. Picture this typical scenario: You've been hiking all day in the rain; your boots are soaked; your socks are soaked. You arrive at your campsite, make camp, and prepare to bed down. Keep in mind that this entire time you've been sloshing around in wet boots. Because you're no longer hiking, your feet are getting cold. Then, when you're all cuddled up in your nice, warm sleeping bag . . . nature calls. Do you really want to put those freezing cold, damp boots on your feet just to make a quick run into the woods?

Another example. It's a wonderful, warm and sunny day and you have to ford a stream. Because of sharp and slick rocks there are very few times when you have the option to remove your boots and cross barefooted. On the other hand, you don't really want to get your boots wet either. A second pair of shoes is a great alternative in this case.

Waldies and Crocs are two brands of clogs popular with A.T. hikers. They are good around camp, but will not stay on your feet for a river crossing. Sandals, such as Teva and similar brands, are also popular and have the benefit of being workable shoes for a river ford. Clogs and sandals are close in terms of weight, so the choice is for comfort, cost, and style.

If you're hiking long distances or thru-hiking, it is not unusual to wear a spare pair of shoes into town to purchase food, wash clothes, etc. These are plenty of good reasons to bring along a second pair of shoes. But choose wisely: the last thing you need is unused dead weight.

SOCKS

It used to be that you needed to wear several pairs of socks with your hiking boots just to be comfortable. Fortunately, the way boots are made now, all you really need is a pair of liner socks and a pair of hiking socks.

Liners are important. They wick away the perspiration and help keep your feet dry. Liners are made of silk, nylon, polypropylene, Thermax, or Orlon. Keep your liners clean. At least rinse them out often so that they don't "clog up" and lose their wicking property. Socks can be hung out to dry on the back of your pack while you walk. You can also use clothespins or safety pins to fasten drying clothes to the back of your pack.

Choose your outer pair of socks wisely. Most experts suggest a blend of wool and nylon or wool and polypropylene. Cotton is never suggested because, unlike wool, it will not keep you warm when it's wet.

Some socks are made with added padding at the toe and heel as well as extra arch support. These socks are usually a nylon-orlon-polypropylene blend; liners are not necessary with them. Try several brands and find out what's right for you. I discovered that mostly wool socks retained too much foot odor for my taste. Frank had absolutely no complaints with his wool-polypropylene blend.

Having frequent changes of socks prevents blisters, and you'll particularly want to change socks during bouts of wet weather. Keep in mind that when you rinse your socks out, you should do it in a bowl or pot and not in a water source (even a stream or lake). Throw the dirty water well away from camp.

BREAKING IN YOUR BOOTS

T he single most important advice when it comes to boots is "break them in." Any experienced hiker will tell you, and it certainly cannot be stressed enough, that boots must be broken in if you intend to hike more than a mile or two in them.

Once you find a pair of boots that fit comfortably on your feet, and you have sealed them properly, then it's time to break them in. Start off by walking around your neighborhood. Wear them to the store and on short errands. If you start to get a blister, don't wait; put Moleskin on it immediately. Catch a hot spot before it becomes a blister and you'll save yourself a lot of pain.

The next step is a day hike. Wear your boots for an entire day, without a pack on your back. If this goes well, you're ready for the final step. If not, continue to day-hike until the boots are comfortable. If you intend to use these boots for more than day hiking, you may want to try hiking with a daypack to see if they are still comfortable with weight on your back. If they are, your boots are ready to go.

Backpacking requires more breaking in time. No matter how comfortable your boots are without a pack that could change once you add 30 or more pounds to your back. A lot of weight on your back changes the way weight is distributed over your feet. And it could change the way your feet feel in your boots. One of the strangest feelings in backpacking is taking your pack off after a long day. Suddenly, it feels as if you're walking on air. If you can backpack a good 5 to 10 miles in your boots without creating any sore spots, your boots are ready for extensive back-packing.

If you are having trouble keeping your feet warm when the temperature drops below freezing, try a vapor barrier. A resealable plastic bag, like those used for packing food, can trap moisture and thus prevent heat from escaping. Place your socked foot into the plastic bag and then slide the bag-wrapped foot into your boot. Though not fashionable, it is cozy.

Chapter Eight

Clothing

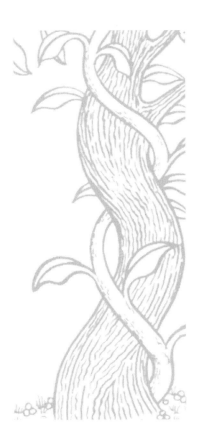

You do not have to carry a backpack full of clothes to be prepared for the types of weather typically found along the Appalachian Trail. Shorts, T-shirts, long johns, pile jackets and pants, and rain gear can be layered to achieve the right combination of warmth and flexibility regardless of the climate. When it comes to backpacking, owning a few high-quality garments will see you through many backpacking trips. Quality and comfort matter much more than style, but often you can have both. One pair of Patagonia shorts, for example, will last as long as, if not longer than, five cheap pairs of shorts. Before discussing the many types of available fabrics, let's look at one of the most critical aspects of backpacking: layering.

LAYERING

Generally, if it's hot and sticky, you won't have to worry about layering—you'll want to strip off as many clothes as you can and still remain decent. When the weather gets cool or cold, you'll need to use layering to ensure you keep warm (or don't overheat).

Layering allows you numerous options, and the clothes involved in layering are lighter, more durable, and allow you greater physical flexibility. The layering system works better than other methods (such as a separate outfit for each weather condition), especially when you get wet or sweat. It is important to layer with the right pieces—long johns, pants or shorts, a pile garment, and a waterproof shell. Layering cotton long johns under blue jeans may keep you warm at first, but as soon as the garments are wet with rain or sweat, you'll be miserable.

When layered correctly, you can easily vent excess warmth. If you begin to sweat, take off your hat first. Because you lose most of your heat through your head, removing your hat or hood will act as a kind of air-conditioning. If you're still hot, unzip your rain-jacket collar and loosen the sleeves (buy rain gear that allows the sleeves to be snugly cinched) to let the air circulate. Remove and add layers as you get warm or cold. It may seem tiresome and time-consuming at the time, but you'll be much more comfortable for the bother.

When preparing for a trip, take the time to select your clothes carefully with layering in mind. Buy an ensemble that can be adjusted to fit the circumstances. Consider your clothing options if you awake to a warm but rainy morning—long johns or shorts, shirt, sweater or fleece jacket, and rain gear. You may want to start out with the shorts, T-shirt, and rain gear; but as it continues to warm up despite the rain, you may drop the rain gear and opt for just getting wet. Later that evening, you pull into camp and, no longer moving, you are likely to get chilled. Pull on your wool sweater and/or your rain gear. If the morning had been rainy and cold instead of warm, a better option would have been long johns under shorts, rain gear, and a hat. Depending on the time of year, you may be comfortable in a pair of loose pants or tights instead of shorts. And one of the better backpacking options is the convertible pant, which offers several options when traveling. Not only are better-quality pants made of quick-dry material but the legs can be zipped off and, voilá, you're wearing shorts. Another zipper along the leg seam allows you to pull the pants legs off over your boots so that you don't have to waste time removing your boots.

A great option for women these days is the sport bra. Many companies make a version of the sports or jog bra that can be worn alone or under a T-shirt so that when things get really hot you can hike in this crop top rather than a heavier T-shirt. Many sports bras are made of CoolMax and wick the sweat away from your body in addition to drying more quickly.

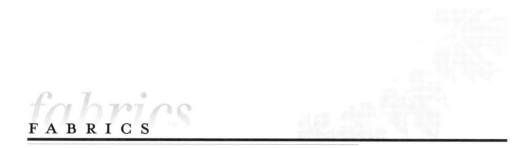

FABRICS

Choosing the fabric of your clothes is as important a decision as choosing what clothes you will bring. But glancing through the pages of an outdoors catalog is a mind-boggling experience! Synthetics with names such as Supplex nylon, Polartec polyester, Thinsulate and Polarguard polyesters, Taslan nylon, Lycra spandex, Cordura nylon, Tactel nylon, Orlon acrylic, Hydrofil nylon, Capilene polyester, and Ultrex nylon make you feel like you need a degree in chemistry to purchase your clothes. Fortunately, it is not as overwhelming as it seems.

ACRYLICS: Fibers polymerized from acrylonitrile are called acrylics and are rarely used in their "pure" form in clothing, except maybe in underwear. Acrylics such as Orlon are often found as a blend, especially in socks. The Orlon adds durability.

COTTON: An ancient fabric with many uses, cotton is an inefficient choice for most outdoor activities. It doesn't keep you warm when it's wet and it takes a long time to dry. For these reasons, cotton clothes that might serve you well at home will not do as well on a backpacking trip. The best example is blue jeans. Not only are they constricting but they double or triple in weight when wet. They also take forever to dry. Other cotton clothing to avoid include long johns, socks, sweaters, and 100-percent cotton T-shirts.

An alternative to 100-percent cotton clothing are trademarked cotton blends. For instance, Patagonia Baggies (shorts) are made of a nylon-cotton blend and are favored by many hikers because they are lightweight, roomy, and water resistant. Many manufacturers make pants and shorts of nylon-cotton blends. T-shirts made of cotton and a synthetic are the most popular hiking shirts because they allow freedom of movement and dry more quickly than all-cotton T-shirts. For day hikes in pleasant weather and moderate altitudes, a cotton T-shirt is a good choice.

DUOFOLD COOLMAX: A unique four-channel design that creates 20 percent more surface area than ordinary fibers, CoolMax ensures fast evaporation, keeping your skin drier. CoolMax comes in a number of different weights for everything from summer to winter wear.

FLEECE: Fleece is a polyester fabric, sometimes constructed with a nylon, Lycra, cotton or ceramic blend, that is generally lightweight and breathable with a high warmth to weight ratio. Some fleeces also have wicking properties.

GORE-TEX: This well-known composite fabric consists of a breathable membrane laminated to various fabrics, which makes them waterproof, windproof, and durable. Stripped-down versions provide only windproofing and breathability. Look carefully at the manufacturer's tag to see which one you are buying.

H2 NO STORM HB: Patagonia's proprietary waterproof, breathable membrane is a three-layer laminate used with fabrics such as nylon or polyester. Primary uses are waterproof, breathable outerwear pieces.

HIND DRYLETE AND ARCTIC DRYLETE: DryLete is an effective moisture-transfer material for a variety of weather conditions. A combination of polyester, hydro-nylon, and Lycra spandex, the fabric rejects sweat as the interior polyester transfers moisture away from your body to the exterior or hydro-nylon, where it can evaporate quickly. It can be both an inner and outer layer. Arctic DryLete is a multitask thermal fabric that siphons perspiration away from the skin. It is made of a soft non-pilling nylon/Lycra knit exterior and a non-pilling, low-pile, polyester-fleece interior.

LYCRA SPANDEX: Lycra is a very stretchy, strong synthetic used extensively in clothing—from cuffs and waistbands on jackets to bras, socks, running tights, and shorts. Tights made of a blend of polypropylene and Lycra are especially popular because they keep you warm and conform to your figure allowing you a lot of freedom of movement.

NYLON: Because it's one of the easiest synthetics to manufacture, you will find many nylons on the market. Nylon is inexpensive, durable, abrasion-resistant, strong, and dries quickly. There are hundreds of types of nylon, from the crinkle-textured Taslan and the supertough Cordura to the supple, softer nylons such as Supplex and ripstop nylon.

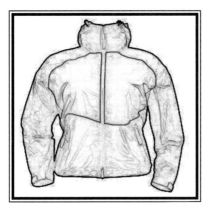

*Midweight shell
(Ground Dash Jacket)*

OMNI-TECH: Columbia's proprietary waterproof, breathable technology is coated or laminated to a nylon or polyester base fabric. Omni-Tech is primarily used for mountaineering, backpacking, and skiing outerwear, as well as an insert in gloves and footwear.

POLARPLUS, POLARLITE, PATAGONIA SYNCHILLA: These bunting or pile materials are good insulators. PolarLite is a lighter and stretchier version of PolarPlus, and Synchilla, Patagonia's well-known double-faced synthetic pile, is bulky and heavy but can be worth the extra bulk and weight on a cold night. For day hikes to higher altitudes, the insulation these materials provide offers good protection from wind and cold when taking a break. The materials are generally far too warm to hike in, but are supposed to be warmer per pound than wool and to dry more quickly than the natural fabric.

POLARTEC CLASSIC: This name applies to vintage Polartec, the product introduced in the 1980s, which revolutionized layering options for outdoor activities. The original still holds its own after repeated washings, and remains a good choice of fabric for backpackers.

POLARTEC WINDBLOC: This is a polyester fabric with a windproof, breathable membrane designed to protect from weather, wind, water, and abrasion.

POLYPROPYLENE: This petroleum-based synthetic is a lightweight fabric that keeps you warm when it's wet. Unlike wool, it dries quickly. When used as first layer of clothing, it keeps your skin dry by transferring moisture to your next layer. Polypropylene is used in long johns and socks. One drawback to polypropylene is that it absorbs the scent of perspiration and must be washed in a special detergent to remove the odor. Polypropylene must be line-dried to prevent shrinkage.

SILK: Silk is one of the lightest fabrics and is often used in long underwear. Although silk is strong and flexible, it tends to be less sturdy than synthetics, giving way at the seams more quickly. It does give you warmth without the bulk, and provides an effective first layer. Silk must be hand-washed and line-dried.

SUPPLEX: Made by DuPont from nylon, Supplex offers the strength and durability of nylon with the supple feel of cotton. It is quick drying, wrinkle resistant, and has the strength to withstand most abrasions, punctures, and tears.

SYMPATEX: Sympatex is a windproof, waterproof, breathable fabric made from nonporous polyester; it is also produced as a nonporous membrane of hydrophilic film that can be laminated onto another fabric. Sympatex comes as three-ply laminates, linings, and inserts for outerwear, footwear, gloves, and other accessories.

THERMAX AND CAPILENE: These synthetics are used in garments that, like polypropylene, draw moisture away from your body to keep you warm. Thermax and Capilene are softer than polypropylene and provide a lot of warmth for their weight. They can be machine washed and tumble dried, and they do not retain perspiration odor.

TRIPLEPOINT CERAMIC: Lowe Alpine System's proprietary waterproof and breathable coating technology, Triplepoint Ceramic is a twin-coated, high-pressure coating that can be applied to a variety of fabrics, including polyester or nylon. The combination of the coating process, fabrics, and durable, water repellent finishes (DWR) all play into the specific windproof, waterproof, or breathable function of each garment.

TYVEK: This high-tech fabric isn't just for house wrap anymore. Some manufacturers use this lightweight, watertight fabric in the manufacture of rain gear.

WOOL: Wool used to be your best bet for winter wear, but it is rapidly being replaced by pile products. The new synthetics—the "Polars" and Synchilla—are giving wool a run for the money. When wool is blended with polypropylene or other synthetics, it makes good socks. Wool keeps you warm when it's wet but it can also be heavy.

TYPES OF CLOTHING

RAIN GEAR

Donning rain gear once meant putting on that heavy rubber yellow slicker, and in some cases the matching pants. In all cases, you felt like a fireman on the way to a three-alarm fire. That, or the Gorton fisherman!

Thankfully, the era of yellow slickers has given way to sophisticated apparel that not only boasts durable waterproof/breathable fabric but also technical design features such as vents, articulated sleeves, and ergonomically correct hoods.

First you must decide what features you need and how much you want to spend before you go to the store. You could easily spend hundreds of dollars on outerwear. A top-of-the-line Gore-Tex jacket can easily cost $400 to $500. Add a pair of pants to your outfit, and you've bought a round-trip ticket to Hawaii.

To narrow the choices, decide if you need a waterproof breathable piece, or simply a jacket that will protect you from the wind and light squalls. The more waterproof a jacket is, the less breathable it is. If you are planning on carrying heavy loads, or are into trail running, you might want to forsake complete water protection for added breathability. Many of the new microfiber fabrics and laminates (of which Gore's Activent is probably the best known) allow for a generous flow of air, protect against wind, and still shed water. They also are softer, lighter, less bulky, and cheaper than most waterproof/breathable shells. There's no sense in forking out big bucks for a waterproof coat if your intention is just to have something lightweight for summer hikes, or simply for blocking a stiff breeze on the trail.

On the other hand, if you plan on hiking the A.T. during winter or early spring/late fall, you should definitely consider a waterproof/breathable model. For four-season use, remember that layering is the name of the game. A heavy-duty shell with a permanent lining is great if you are expecting arctic weather, but is too heavy and hot for most hiking activities. Your best bet is a shell with a zip-out liner, or simply a shell that is large enough to accommodate a fleece jacket or wool sweater underneath. However, sometimes you just want to put on a warm jacket without a bunch of layers. The insulated shell may not be as versatile, but it can be more convenient in cold weather.

One cautionary note—the new Windbloc or Windstopper fleece apparel is great for a top layer, but inappropriate for a second layer under a waterproof/breathable shell. Since the windblocking material trades breathability for wind management, it works like a sweat chamber if layered under another not-so-breathable garment.

You may wonder if you need rain gear at all, especially if you hike during the summer. In warm weather, hikers often refuse to fight the battle, opting to get wet by hiking in the rain in just shorts and T-shirt. That's all well and good when it's steamy outside, but when the temperature drops (which it can do even in the summer), you risk hypothermia. A shell, waterproof or windproof, will help retain heat and guard against hypothermia, making rain gear is one of the most essential items on your clothing checklist.

WHAT TO LOOK FOR IN RAIN GEAR

One of the most popular names in rain gear of late is Frogg Toggs, a less-expensive (though less-durable) alternative to Gore-Tex products. They are not widely available through outdoor retailers, but you can view their online catalog at **www.frogg toggs.com.** We know of one hiker who has thru-hiked the Trail three times using their gear.

Tyvek aside, the most common name in shell material is Gore-Tex, the fabric of choice for most brands of rain gear. It is also true that you will pay more money for the designer label. There are also literally dozens of similar fabrics, such as Sympatex, Triplepoint Ceramic, Omni-Tech, and H2 No Storm HB, that offer relatively similar performance.

Rather than asking for a Gore-Tex jacket when you walk into the store, tell the clerk you are interested in a waterproof/breathable shell. Gore-Tex should be one of your options, but if it is the only thing you are shown, go to another store. Rather than sweat the manufacturer of the waterproof/breathable laminate or coating on the fabric, focus on features instead. Check articles for meticulously taped seams with no bumps or bubbles, perfect stitching, and a good fit.

One advantage to buying a Gore-Tex or Sympatex jacket is that both companies mandate that manufacturers who use their products make sure that the garments adhere to a minimum standard of performance. All rain-gear DWR finishes will eventually wear off. When this happens, you can apply products like Nikwax, ReviveX, or Zepel to restore the finish. You'll know you have lost your DWR when the coat appears to be absorbing water. It is not the fault of the waterproof/breathable membrane but results from the DWR finish no longer causing water to bead on the fabric's surface.

Sorting out the drawbacks and advantages of three-ply versus two-ply shells is worse than the debate over whether 2000 or 2001 was the first year of the new millennium. The systems work the same, but three-ply usually costs more. Two-ply jackets have a mesh lining, which adds weight but may move easier when layered over fleece or wool.

Don't forget to check the jacket's warranty. Some companies, like The North Face, offer a lifetime warranty on the product—your lifetime, not the coat's. Make sure the company from which you are buying guarantees the jacket will live up to its advertised performance.

If you are female, keep in mind that there are an increasing number of "woman-specific" jackets on the market. These coats are cut shorter in the sleeves and torso, wider in the hips, and narrower in the shoulders than men's/unisex models. You can expect the same features and durability from a women's jacket as a men's design; however, many companies don't make their top-of-the-line performance coats in anything but men's small, medium, and large. Although a women's model may fit you better (as it could a small-framed man), don't limit your selection to women's only. Women with large shoulders and a more athletic build might well find a better fit in a unisex model, so take advantage of the opportunity to try on all available styles.

HOODS

The weakest link of most jackets is hood design. Look for a model that will tuck away when not needed, so you don't always have it flapping in the breeze. Zip-off hoods are an option, especially if you don't plan on using the hood. However, you run the risk of reaching for it in a downpour and realizing you left it in a drawer back home. A common downfall of hoods is that they cut off peripheral vision and hinder breathing when they are zipped into position. A well-designed hood should swivel when you turn your head and allow for adequate breathing space when zipped. Check the adjustment straps on the hood. Will your hair get caught in the toggle cords? Can you see out of the face hole when the hood is up, or do you feel like a turtle peering out of its shell?

VENTILATION

Anyone who has walked uphill knows how fast you can work up a sweat. The fabric of your jacket may breathe better than a good Pinot Noir, but you'll still need built-in vents to accommodate the heat you create during rigorous activity. The most common ventilation systems are underarm vent zips that, when opened, allow warm air out and cool air in. "Pit zips" are a priority feature on waterproof/breathable jackets but less important on shells designed only to thwart wind. Many companies still persist in overkill closure measures for pit zips by adding a Velcro flap over the zipper. Unfortunately, the Velcro inevitably sticks shut when you want it open, defeating the vent's purpose. Look for a coat with sealed zippers and no Velcro.

To test the workability of a pit zip, grab the tip of your left jacket sleeve by the fingers of your left hand. Stretch your arm above your head, keeping a hold of the sleeve. With your right arm, reach over, grab the zipper, and open or close the vent. If the zipper doesn't slide easily with this single-hand method, look for another coat. Some jacket designs come with chest zips and mesh-lined pockets, both of which add ventilation. The advantage of chest zips is that they are convenient to open and allow quick access to the breast pockets of your second layer of clothes. The downside is that they can be mistaken for pockets themselves, which can lead to lost car keys and wallets.

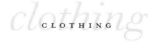

Lately, manufacturers have been making increasing use of back and chest yokes for ventilation. While these always-open flaps (sometimes with a mesh inner lining) do provide additional breathability, they aren't appropriate for cold weather or high-wind use, since they can't be sealed shut.

OTHER RAINCOAT FEATURES

One design feature you might find when searching for rain gear is the crotch straps on the bottom of the waterproof/breathable jacket. Obviously this is to keep it from pulling out of your rain pants. Is it comfortable? We don't think so but if you don't mind that type of thing it may be a plus for you. Here are some other features to check out:

- If your jacket of choice has a drawcord at the waist, check to make sure it doesn't interfere with the waist belt of your pack.

- Check the durability of the zippers. Large-tooth zippers seem to hold up better than standard coil zippers. It is interesting that recently, Gore did alter its standards to accommodate new waterproof zipper technology, which is now available on Arc'teryx and Wild Things jackets.

- Scrutinize the zipper pull and end tangs for reinforcements, as these areas are the most likely points of failure.

- Look at the cuffs on the coat. Velcro closures here are good because they can be tightened to seal out water or worn loose for added breathability and comfort.

- Bring along any and all accouterments you might be wearing with your coat—packs, harnesses, gloves, and secondary layers. Your jacket will ideally be part of a system that will keep you warm, dry, and comfortable, so make sure all components work together to meet that goal.

PONCHOS/UMBRELLAS

The least effective of all rain-gear options, most backpacking ponchos are designed to cover both you and your pack. Ponchos do shield you from a lot of the rain under ideal conditions, but in the wind they are practically useless. While a minority of hikers find that ponchos meet their needs, most hikers who have tried ponchos dispose of them during their hike.

And yes, you will probably run into those happy few who are content to sing in the rain as long as they have an umbrella over their head. Some people highly recommend umbrellas, particularly Ray Jardine, author of *Beyond Backpacking.* Jardine even offers instructions for umbrella modifications in his book. He and his wife, Jenny, won't leave home without theirs, and recommend not using them only in fierce storms and gale-force winds.

HATS

Hats are an indispensable part of your backpacking outfit because much of the body's heat is lost through your head. If your feet are cold, put on a hat. Warming your head will do more toward warming your feet than adding an extra pair of socks. Another pair of socks might actually make your feet colder by making your boots too tight and constricting the circulation in your feet.

A wool cap with a polypropylene liner will keep your head warm while wicking away perspiration. Thermax hats are also good for the same reason. If you will be doing a lot of cold-weather backpacking, you may want to invest in a balaclava. This stretchy hat covers your head and neck and most of your face and is much lighter to carry than an extra shirt or sweater!

While not as warm, baseball-style caps are great for keeping the sun off your head and face. They are also great worn under your rain jacket hood, keeping the hood from dripping rain on your nose and helping the hood move with your head. All types of baseball caps are available, including those that offer a neck flap for extra protection against the sun.

For those of you who go for the high-tech products, Sequel offers the Desert Rhat Hat. An adjustable chin strap keeps the hat on your head even in high winds; a large bill with a black underbrim provides sun protection for your eyes and face; a breathable lining of Tex-O-Lite metallic film shields the top of your head from the sun's intensity; a removable white cape reflects the sun; and a terrycloth headband absorbs the sweat.

GLOVES

My hands get cold easily but I find that when hiking I rarely need gloves. Cold, wet days are the worst once you make camp. I've used glove liners without the gloves fairly successfully—they are easier to maneuver your fingers in because they don't have the bulk of leather gloves. But for those days when sticking your hands in your pockets just won't do (what if you take a tumble with your hands in your pockets?), there are a number of glove/mitten options available. From Gore-Tex shell and wool mittens to gloves of wool, wool-blends, Thinsulate, pile, and other synthetics, you should be able to find a pair of hand warmers that fits your needs.

Keep in mind that you can also purchase glove and mitten liners (usually very lightweight and made of silk or synthetics used in the manufacture of thermal underwear) for extracold days. If you're desperate, use plastic bags as vapor barrier–style gloves.

BANDANAS

In the backpacking world, you're not a true hiker unless you have at least one bandana on your person. Bandanas are wonderfully versatile. I use them as headbands, hats, and handkerchiefs. They can also be used to strain water before filtering and to cool hot necks (dipping the bandana in water and loosely tying about your throat). Similarly, they can be used as a cloth for washing or as a towel for drying (your body and your dishes). I always carry several with me when I am backpacking.

GAITERS

Hiking gaiters are made of water-resistant materials. They fasten below the knee and extend to cover the upper portion of your boots. Their purpose is to keep water and snow out of your boots so that they remain dry.

Gaiters come in a variety of heights, from ankle-height to just below the knee. Some hikers wear the ankle gaiters to keep dust and leaves from working their way into their boots or running shoes. Gaiters are also useful when you hike through wet brush, grass, leaves, and poison ivy.

Unlike pack covers and rain gear, gaiters are not essential rainwear for any hike. However, they may make your hike more comfortable and are worth looking into, particularly for hikes in the snow.

TOWN CLOTHES

If you intend to spend more than a week on the Trail, and especially if you're going to be long-distance hiking, you may want to consider bringing along a set of

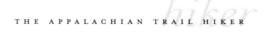

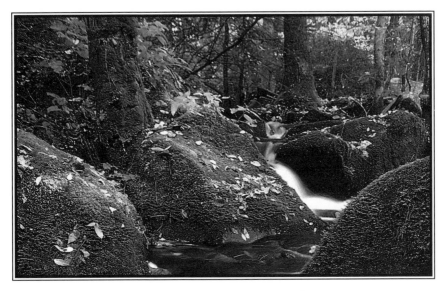

A cold stream in Great Smoky Mountains National Park

"town clothes." All this means is that you stash away one shirt that you will wear only when hitching or hiking into a town. Your appearance and your attitude will determine how you are treated when you go to town. Some female hikers carry broomstick gauze skirts. They can pack down small, they're light, and they're supposed to look wrinkled anyway.

TAKING CARE OF CLOTHING

While backpacking, care of your clothing will be limited to a bit of rinsing here and there. On short trips (unless your clothes get really awful), you can wait with cleaning your clothing until you get home.

While hiking, I rinse out my nylon shorts every day or every other day, depending on the sweat factor. I simply rinse them in a cookpot and hang them to dry on a branch or rock if it's a dry night. If it's wet outside, I take them to bed with me, stuffing them at the bottom of my sleeping bag. If they are not dry by morning, I just wait for body heat to dry them out while I hike (or wet them down again with my sweat).

T-shirts and socks can be rinsed in the same manner and cleaned once a week (use a biodegradable soap only when necessary). Some synthetics require a special detergent to rid them of their perspiration odors. Read labels and know before you go. Never wash your clothes in a water source—even biodegradable soaps leave suds and a bad taste. Always dump dirty wash water far from any water source. If you are on a long-distance hike, you will hit an occasional town where you can wash your clothes in a laundromat.

Another method for drying clothes—other than hanging them on a branch or rock—is by using your rope to form a clothesline. Lightweight clothes pins are available at outdoors stores or you can center your rope around a tree, twist it tightly, tie it to another tree, and then pull apart a twist to hold your clothes. You may want to carry a thin, lightweight line just for this purpose. Also, it is not uncommon on the trail to see clothes, particularly socks, hanging from the back of a pack as they dry.

VAPOR-BARRIER SYSTEM

A vapor-barrier system is a quick way to get warm when you're really cold. The barrier can be a Mylar "space blanket" or a less exotic, impermeable barrier such as a plastic bag that will retain both your body's heat and moisture. Although not exactly comfortable, because you stay wet, it is extremely effective in capturing body heat.

Vapor barriers can be used in sleeping-bag liners and in clothes such as pants, shirts, socks, and gloves. We think vapor barriers are just fine when it's freezing cold outside and there is no other way to get warm. We have used plastic bags a number of times to warm up our feet, especially when our boots have failed to dry from the previous day's rain and it is raining again.

Some people believe in using vapor barriers in all cold-weather situations, while others would rather die (or so they say) than submit themselves to the agony of the vapor barrier.

Try vapor-barrier liners before you decide. You may like the specialty gear or you may decide it's not worth carrying the garments and that you would rather rely on Ziploc bags for the occasional need for extra warmth.

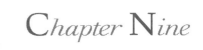
Other Equipment

In addition to the basics—tent, pack, boots, sleeping bag, etc.—there are some other articles you will want to consider taking on a hike, especially if you're out for a night or more. Carefully select the equipment you really need, and leave at home things that are unnecessary or redundant. You will be more comfortable without the added weight.

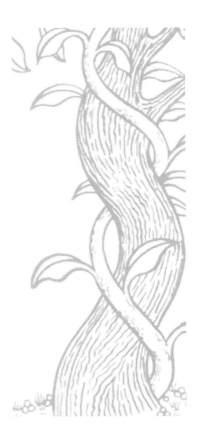

LIGHTING

lighting

Very simply, it is a good idea to bring along some source of light for evenings at camp and on the trail. From time to time, it will be a relief to have a light to help find things in a dark tent or shelter. Even if you are day-hiking, a light can help you find your way should you end up hiking in the dark.

HEADLAMPS

Hands free operation is a big plus for all sorts of camp chores. This is the chief advantage headlamps have over candle lanterns and other flashlights. You can cook, clean, and set up your tent without having to set your flashlight down. Though not recommended, if you're seriously into night hiking, then you have another good reason to look into purchasing a headlamp. These illuminators light the way ahead of you for approximately 30 feet. But they, too, use batteries and have a few other drawbacks, as well.

Headlamps have two basic designs—either with the lamp and batteries attached to the headband or with the lamp attached to the headband and the battery unit (sometimes including yet another light) attached to a belt and connected to the headband by wire. The problem with the all-in-one unit is that it tends to be heavy and to induce headaches if you use it for long periods of time. The problem with the latter is that the wires can get caught by branches, arms, etc., or short-out due to nicks or complete severing. A couple of advantages to the two-part system are that it reduces headlamp headaches and, when kept on your person, the batteries stay warm when it's cold—a chief drainer of battery energy.

One important factor to keep in mind when carrying a headlamp is that battery switches tend to come on while sitting in your pack. Unless your headlamp's design guards against this, you need to make sure your headlamp remains in the off position while packed away.

Depending on your needs, there are a number of functional LED headlamps available. A few safe bets for lighting are the Petzl Tikka+, Petzl Myo, Princeton Tec Scout, Princeton Tec Yukon, and the Hartford Easter Seals HL-4AA, sometimes sold as a store brand, are your best bets. Your choice will depend on how you want to factor weight, ease of use, lighting needs, and price.

One ultralight option is the Q Lighting Bil-Light Sul a one-ounce light that clips to the bill of your hat. While it won't illumine the path for night hiking, it does offer sufficient candlepower for reading, journaling, cooking, and organizing your gear in the dark.

FLASHLIGHTS

The flashlight you take backpacking needn't be really powerful. Most hikers use the smaller flashlights equipped with a lithium battery or even a couple of alkaline AA batteries. They are small but adequate. Mini Maglites are popular with hikers because they provide a lot of candle power for very little weight. Another hot item is the tiny Pak-Lite mini LED, which only weighs 1.5 ounces and runs 1,200 hours on low output and 200 hours at its brightest setting. The tiny light unit snaps onto the end of a 9-volt battery, which doubles as the light's body.

Flashlights that require two D cell batteries, or more, are too heavy even for overnight hikes, and the illumination is overkill for what you'll need when hiking. Remember, though, no matter which flashlight you pick, you will need a ready supply of batteries for longer hikes.

LANTERNS

Big, heavy, white-gas lanterns have a place in camping but not in backpacking. They are bright and efficient but are far too heavy and bulky to carry along on a backpacking trip. There are also heavy battery-powered lanterns that weigh even more and are made for family camping.

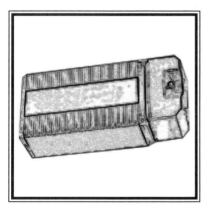

Pak-Lite Mini LED

Two lightweight lanterns to consider are the Primus Micron Lantern and the Snow Peak Gigapower Lantern, which each weigh in at 4.5 ounces. Brunton manufactures a mantleless lantern (8.3 ounces) that screws onto a butane canister. It features piezo ignition without priming. The same caution regarding stoves in the tent can be extended to stove-style lanterns. Make sure the tent is well ventilated if you use one inside it.

Candle lanterns are another good option for lighting. We started out on our first backpacking trip with one, and have continued to use ours, although we have long since added a flashlight. Candle lanterns weigh as little as six ounces (sold by Limelight Productions, REI, Early Winters, and at some outdoors stores under the generic Candle Lantern). One candle will give you as much as eight hours of illumination. The light produced by a candle lantern is not very bright, though in a crunch it can substitute for a flashlight to use while cooking, cleaning, reading, or writing when you make camp at dark.

The candle lantern is safer than a candle. The candle is housed inside metal and glass, so you are less likely to start a fire if it tips over. A lanterned candle is also more efficient because it is protected from the wind and, thus, does not burn as quickly as a lone candle. You can purchase a candle lantern for $10 to $20; candle refills are about 50 cents.

Other possibilities are small oil and gas lanterns, which burn up to 20 hours per fill-up. These units cost about $20 to $25 and weigh the same as candle lanterns. Some of these lanterns can take different grades of lamp oil, including citronella (the insect repellent).

All lanterns are equipped with a hanger and can often be rigged to hang from the apex of your tent by an attached nylon cord. Many tents have loops in the apex that will allow you to fasten a cord. If your tent does not have a loop at its apex, it may be possible to add a loop of Velcro or sew on a loop, yourself. Some tents have loops in the corners designed to hold gear lofts from which you can rig a line to hold a candle lantern. Remember to keep the lantern a safe distance from the material of the tent so you won't burn holes in the tent or set it afire.

TOILETRIES

D epending on the length of your hiking trip, you may want to consider bringing along items such as towel, shampoo/soap, deodorant, razors/shaving cream, toothbrush/toothpaste, eyecare items, and toilet paper.

Towel

Most hikers do not carry a towel, per se. We usually carry bandanas and one handcloth for the purpose of washing and/or drying. In warm weather, we let the sun do the job of drying our skin. In cold weather, we use the cloth to hand bathe ourselves with heated water and then dry with a bandana.

For those who need a towel, the super absorbent Cascade Designs Pack-Towl is available. The manufacturer boasts the towel can absorb up to ten times its weight as well as dry quickly (which is important because who wants to carry around a soggy, one-pound towel). Most outdoors stores offer this towel and other variations such as the MSR PackTowl.

Shampoo/Soap

Some folks have no qualms about getting dirty and sweaty on the trail, waiting until they are back home or to a hotel, campground, or hostel until cleaning up. For those who prefer to keep clean while on the trail, there are a number of shampoos/soaps options.

Biodegradable soap, such as Dr. Bronner's, can't be beat for washing your body, and is the preferred choice because it impacts the environment less than other soaps. These soaps, though, do not work well as a shampoo, leaving your hair lank and greasy. Before depending on a biodegradable soap as an all-round cleaner, I would suggest testing it on the various things you plan to use it for, such as hair, body, clothes, pots, and pans, to see how you like it. There are a number of other biodegradable soaps available from outdoors stores, including Mountain Suds, Bio-suds, and Sunshower Soap.

There is a soap product on the market called NO-Rinse that requires no water for a shampoo and only one quart of water to bathe. N/R Laboratories claims that you simply massage NO-Rinse in and towel dry it out.

If your soap doesn't work as a shampoo, most discount department stores (such as Wal-Mart and K-Mart) and drug stores offer trial or sample size products that are great for backpacking. Shampoos are commonly available in sample sizes as are toothpastes and lotions. I've used a variety of shampoos while backpacking but if you can find a biodegradable shampoo you'll lessen your detrimental effect on the environment.

A lot of the water sources along trails provide drinking water for hikers as well as for animals, so as with any soaps, never wash your hair or body in or near a water source. Would you want to drink soapy water freshly rinsed from a fellow hiker's sweaty body?

DEODORANT

While soap is a necessity, deodorant is considered optional. We use it only on visits to town. Otherwise, there's no one around to smell you but yourself (and other smelly hikers)! You may also want to consider that the less smelly you are, in terms of artificial odors such as perfumed deodorants, the less likely you'll be to scare wildlife away or to attract unwanted insects.

The most natural way to deodorize yourself is by using a deodorant rock. Composed of natural mineral salts, this crystal-like deodorant supposedly lasts a full year with normal use. Deodorant rocks are available at health food stores and through some catalogs. Two of the more popular brands are NATURE'S Pure Crystal Deodorant and Le Crystal's Naturel.

Another relatively natural way to deodorize yourself is to use a baking soda-based powder such as Shower to Shower. Victoria's father has used it successfully for years. If you're not interested in these natural methods of stopping perspiration odor, you can always carry your favorite deodorant in its sample or regular size.

Do keep in mind, especially during the hot and humid days of summer, that you probably reek. Fortunately, the longer you're out on the trail, deodorant-less, the more you become accustomed to your body's odor, which, believe it or not, isn't half as bad as the odor perspiration leaves in your clothes. So if you intend on hitchhiking into town to resupply, you might want to consider tidying up yourself. Give a quick wash under your arms and change into clean clothes. People will be more willing to give needy hikers a hitch if they look presentable and smell as inoffensive as possible.

While staying with some friends during one backpacking trip we left a lasting impression on our hostess's olfactory nerves. She later told us that on our first night there she had prowled about the house, sniffing, unable to sleep or to determine the cause of the ungodly smell. Finally she stepped into the entranceway and found the odoriferous source of her nocturnal wanderings—our boots! She quickly banished them outdoors. Embarrassing? You betchum Red Rider. When someone offers you hospitality while backpacking, the last thing you want to do is offend them. If someone invites you to stay, kindly leave your boots outside. Remember, you're used to their smell, but others will find it overwhelming. Most people will be too polite to mention it, so it's up to you to keep your odor under control, at least when you're off the Trail.

One of the worst ways hikers offend people is by dining in restaurants when they are dirty. The Appalachian Trail Conservancy has actually received complaints about this and some restaurants have lost business. They may love your business, but think about it. . . would you really enjoy eating a meal in your hometown if some smelly, unwashed person came in and sat down in the booth behind you? Use some common courtesy when eating in restaurants, clean yourself up a bit, and change into a clean shirt at the very minimum. Also, leave your pack outside, if you can. Your pack, like your boots, can smell as bad as you do!

RAZORS/SHAVING CREAM

Most men opt to grow a beard when hiking, although some do take the trouble to shave every day or now and then. The same goes for women—many prefer to let the hair under their arms and on their legs grow out while hiking. It's all a matter of preference. When long-distance hiking, we shave at least once a week, using biodegradable soap and a disposable razor, because we are more comfortable that way. A battery-operated electric razor is another option.

TOOTHBRUSH AND TOOTHPASTE

Just as you shouldn't wash your hair near a water source, please don't brush your teeth near one either. Dig a small hole at least 200 feet away from water sources to spit into and then cover your spit.

As for toothcare products, there are a variety of options on the market, but a child's toothbrush works great because it is small and lightweight! Toothpaste can easily be purchased in sample sizes or you might want to try using baking soda that you can transfer to a small bottle for convenience. If you can live without toothpaste, do so. If you use dental floss, please pack it out.

EYECARE

We are continually amazed at the number of hikers who elect to wear contact lenses during their long-distance hikes. But as risky as it seems, Victoria wears contacts; although she carries a pair of glasses, just in case. The new, disposable, daily- and extended-wear lenses are easy to care for, and the cleaning fluid does not add much weight to her pack. Personally, unless she is sitting still, her body heat raised by the exertion of hiking, fogs her glasses up so badly, they're useless. And, when she's sweaty they tend to slide off her nose.

These days you don't even have to worry if you can't get your hands clean enough to remove your contacts. There are several products available now, such as Purell Instant Hand Sanitizer, that allow you to clean your hands by rubbing them with an antiseptic gel cleanser. Just make sure you wait a few seconds for the alcohol to dry before handling your lenses. The gel, which is flammable, can also be used in an emergency to start a fire.

TOILET PAPER AND TROWEL

One of the worst sights we saw while hiking through the Great Smoky Mountains were the wads of toilet paper scattered through the woods near shelters. Of course backpackers need to bring toilet paper, and even day hikers need it occasionally, but all hikers should dispose of their waste and toilet paper properly.

When you do have to go, never relieve yourself near a water source. Always find a site at least 200 feet downhill or to the side of a water source, campsite, shelter, or trail. Dig a cathole about six to eight inches deep and, if possible, keep the top layer of soil and root fibers intact, so it can be returned to the spot in one relatively undisturbed piece. When you are done, stir in dirt with a stick, cover with at least two inches of soil, and camouflage the cathole. This is for the protection of wildlife as well as other hikers. According to the Centers for Disease Control and Prevention, beavers living downstream from national parks and forests contract giardiasis (caused by humans) more often than humans do.

A good way to pack toilet paper is to scrunch it flat and stick it in a resealable plastic bag. By removing the cardboard tube in the center and unraveling the paper from the inside, you will find that your toilet paper crushes down flatter in its plastic bag. Scot toilet tissue seems to have the most paper for the money. Though you can dig a hole with a stick, a backpacker's trowel weighs a mere two ounces and costs next to nothing. That's well worth the "trouble" when you consider how much it will lessen your environmental impact. Packing out the paper is not absolutely essential but it sure is a great way to taken an extra step toward lessening your environmental impact.

Digging a hole with your boot heel doesn't dig a deep enough hole easily and it disturbs the environment more than necessary. A lightweight plastic trowel (usually about two ounces) made for backpacking is an important Leave-No-Trace tool for hikers. The U-Dig-It hand shovel is the Hummer-like option, which is quite heavy-duty for its 6.5 ounces. A third option is to use a wide metal tent stake.

Always wash your hands after defecating, whether it is briskly rubbing your hands together under water or using an antibacterial hand gel. Your partner can pour water over your hands or you can pour your own with the bottle grasped between your knees. To keep yourself healthy (or at least give your health a fighting chance), refrain from sharing foods such as gorp, because viruses can easily be passed from hiker to hiker this way.

A note to women: Urination for male backpackers is as easy, if not easier because there is no seat to lift, as it is in the "real" world. And although some trails offer the occasional outhouse, the chances of stumbling upon one at the appropriate moment are about nil. Even then, you're likely to find a note requesting you to relieve yourself in the woods because some outhouses are reserved for defecation only.

If you're strong enough and have a good aim, it is possible to pee with your pack on—release the hipbelt, drop your drawers to your knees, bend your knees a bit, lean forward with your hands on your knees for support, relax, and go.

Another option is take off your pack and find what Kathleen Meyer, author of *How to Shit in the Woods,* calls the perfect pose. Find two rocks, a rock and a log, two logs, or if necessary, a steep slope and a log or rock. Sitting on one, you balance your feet on the other and avoid the splashed boots that are so common when women try to pee outdoors.

A third option is a funnel, but make sure you purchase one with a long hose. The funnels are designed to slip easily into your pants and transport your urine outside. Victoria never got up the nerve to try hers, feeling certain that no matter what she did she'd end up with soggy britches.

Menstruation is another problem women face in the wilderness. On most trips, it's going to be "pack it in, pack it out;" so make sure you bring along enough resealable bags to hold your used tampons or napkins.

Your best choice is going to be an applicatorless tampon such as OBs. They are compact and produce the least amount of waste all the way around. Once used, wrap them in a bit of toilet paper and seal in a plastic bag until you reach a suitable dumping station. Never drop your tampons or napkins into a latrine nor bury them, because it will take them years to disintegrate, if animals don't dig them up first.

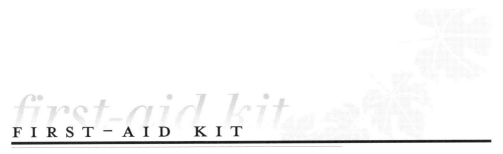

FIRST-AID KIT

K eeping in mind that it is next to impossible to create a perfect first-aid kit, the following is a list of what makes up a close-to-perfect kit:

- A Ziploc or other brand zipper-lock plastic bag to hold the items in your first-aid kit

- Approximately six 1 x 3-inch band-aids. These can be used to cover most scratches, cuts, and scrapes.

- Two 4 x 4-inch sterile gauze pads that can be cut down or doubled up depending on the size of the wound

- A roll of athletic tape—one inch by ten yards—has a variety of uses from holding on the sterile gauze to wrapping ankles.

- Tincture of benzoin. Not only does this liquid toughen feet but it helps tape stick better when rubbed on the skin.

- A couple of butterfly band-aids for closing small, gaping wounds

- An individually wrapped sanitary napkin is great for stanching heavily bleeding wounds.

- Povidone-iodine ointment has a number of uses: disinfects wounds (straight from the tube); dissolves in water for a wash for larger scrapes; and can even be used as a lubricant or to treat water in an emergency.

- Moleskin or some other padding to treat hot spots and blisters

- Your favorite painkiller for aches, pains, fever, etc.

- A six-inch-wide elastic wrap (such as an Ace wrap). These can be used to wrap strains and sprains as well as to hold bandages in place, constrict snakebites, compress heavy bleeding, or splint a broken bone.

- A few safety pins always come in handy. They can also hold an Ace bandage, drain blisters, repair clothing, and more.

- A few antihistamine tablets, such as Benadryl, to combat insect bites and poison ivy.

- Pepto-bismol and Imodium or some similar tablets for upset stomachs.

- A mirror to check for ticks (if you don't hike with a partner)

- Scissors and tweezers. (You may be able to find a pocketknife with these items. My Victorinox has both and they have come in handy many times.)

Other items to consider, depending on the time of year and the location of your hike, are meat tenderizer or Sting-eze for insect bites, sunscreen, alcohol to rub on and and toughen feet, lip balm, lotion, prescription drugs if you need them, a bee sting kit if you are allergic to insect stings, and DEET repellent for mosquitoes and other insects. Remember that a first-aid kit is a very personal thing. For example, if you have trouble with constipation at home, by all means carry a laxative while hiking.

I use lip balm (Chap Stick works best for me) constantly both at home and while hiking. I can't abide the feeling of chapped lips and always carry several tubes of Chap Stick with me. Other good lip balms are Blistex, Carmex, and Labiosin. You can find many options both at drug stores and outdoors stores.

Some people have problems with hemorrhoids while hiking, and always include Preparation H or Tucks Pads in their kits. Some women may find it necessary to carry birth-control pills.

Hiking in the summer, desert, or snow might make it necessary for you to carry a sunscreen with a sun protection factor (SPF) in line with your skin's sensitivity to the sun. The higher the SPF, the less likely you are to be burned. As with lip balms, you can find a wide range of sunscreens to choose from at your local drug, discount, and outdoors stores.

Lotion is another product you may wish to add to your kit if you intend to be hiking in hot, dry weather. Some sunscreens combine lotion with the screen or you may wish to carry a sample size of your favorite brand. Remember, though, that baby oil acts as a sun tan lotion as well as a skin softener and could be potentially dangerous if you intend to use it as a lotion.

But, unless you have a special need or problem, do not carry too many specific items in your first-aid kit. The kit and its contents should be as versatile as possible. It won't matter that you have to cover a two-inch-wide wound with a four-inch-wide bandage, for example.

Also, remember to repack your first-aid kit seasonally or yearly. Medicines expire and may need to be replaced so always check the expiration dates before heading out on any trip. And there is no use carrying insect repellent on a winter trip when there are no bugs around. Your first-aid kit should reflect your personal needs as well as the season and geographic area through which you're hiking.

Most importantly, do not carry anything in your kit that you do not know how to use. For example, a suture kit will be useless to you unless you have been trained in suturing wounds. Don't carry prescription medicines unless you are fully aware of their effects and how to use them.

Depending on how safety-conscious you are, there are all sorts of items available to ease your mind while hiking. Everything from dental emergency kits to accident report forms can be purchased for your first-aid kit.

Although I've never known any one to use one, some people feel safer if they carry along a snakebite kit. There are several kits on the market ranging from $5 to $15. The simplest kit contains two big suction cups plus a smaller suction cup for bites on small surfaces such as fingers. The kit also includes a lymph constrictor, scalpel, antiseptic vial, and instructions. The $10 Extractor is a double-chamber vacuum pump with four cup sizes, antiseptic, band-aids, a safety razor, instructions, and a carrying case. Whether these snakebite kits actually work is debatable. In any case, get a snakebite victim to medical care as soon as possible.

Outdoors stores offer a variety of first-aid kits ranging in price from $8 to $80. Outdoor Research, Adventure Medical Kits, and REI are some of the major manufacturers of first-aid kits.

No matter which kit you choose, the items will be more useful if you take a wilderness first aid, or a first responder course by a group such as SOLO (**www.soloschools.com**) or NOLS (**www.nols.edu**).

ITEMS FOR EMERGENCIES

When it comes to emergencies, some people like to carry along a mirror, flares, and a whistle. Victoria carries a mirror anyway, because she needs it to insert her contact lenses, but you may want to consider carrying a mirror should you need it to signal someone below or above you. If your watch has a reflective surface you can discard the mirror and use your watch instead. Some compasses have sighting mirrors that can be used for signaling, or you can use foil, your stove's windscreen (if it reflects), or even your sunglasses. Signal mirrors, on the other hand, are usually too heavy to be carried by a backpacker.

We've never carried one, but some backpackers feel safer if they carry along a flare or smoke bomb for emergencies. The bombs emit clouds of orange or red smoke that can be seen from both the ground and the air. Flares can be shot up into the air and usually burn for an average of seven seconds. We have seen both smoke bombs and flares available through catalogs—$8 for the bomb, $16 for three flares—and most outdoors stores keep them in stock as well.

For use in both an emergency and as a warning to bears, you can also carry a whistle in your "emergency kit." Just make sure you use the whistle only in emergency situations because in addition to crying "wolf," you'll also be disturbing other people out there who are seeking peace and quiet. If you purchase a whistle, make sure the balls inside are made of metal or plastic. Cork, if it gets wet, will ruin your whistle. Survival whistles can be purchased for under $3. Three blasts are a recognized distress signal, as a short form of the three short, three long, three short blasts of an SOS cry.

There is a gadget on the market called the Survivo II that includes an accurate compass, waterproof matchcase, whistle, striking flint, and signal mirror. It is packed in a 4.5 x 1.25-inch case and weighs a mere ounce.

SUNGLASSES

There are so many options when it comes to sunglasses that I cannot begin to recommend any one particular brand. If you do carry sunglasses, make sure that the lenses are designed to filter out the sun's harmful rays—both ultraviolet and infrared. Sunglasses are especially essential for snow hiking where the sun reflects off the ground and into your eyes.

Sunglasses can be purchased for as little or as much as you want to spend. Straps to hold your sunglasses around your neck—Chums, Croakies, and others—are worth the extra money because they keep you from losing your them. This is especially beneficial if you just paid a lot of money for your shades.

There are also a number of other "gadgets" that can be purchased for sunglasses (and glasses, if you wear them) including defoggers, lens cleaners, cases, windguards, and clip-on sunshades for eyeglass wearers.

Sunglasses are now manufactured for children, including glasses that filter out ultraviolet and infrared rays.

SUNSCREEN

Walking in shorts and a T-shirt leaves a hiker exposed to the suns rays for several hours a day. To prevent burning, wear a sunscreen or sunblock. If you have fair or sensitive skin, you will need a sunscreen with a sun protection factor (SPF) of at least 15; the higher the SPF, the greater the protection.

BATTERIES

When it comes to backpacking, there are only two types of batteries that are worth considering—alkaline and lithium. Whichever source you opt for, you'll be happier if all the battery-powered devices you carry use the same type of battery. This simplifies carrying extras.

ALKALINE: These batteries are far more efficient and longer-lasting than carbon-zinc batteries. They offer as much as double the life yet weigh and cost just a bit more. Unlike carbon-zinc cells, the alkaline battery dies suddenly rather than fades out—a minor disadvantage. Alkaline batteries do revive themselves a bit naturally (without a charger) and will last for another 20 minutes or so if left to rest for half-a-day unlike standard batteries that recharge only enough to put out a dim light for another five minutes. Alkaline cells cost about $2.50 for two AA batteries, $3 for two C batteries, and $3 for two D batteries.

LITHIUM: Extremely light and efficient, lithium batteries are also expensive (though in ratio to their effectiveness and weight not inordinately so). Topping alkaline batteries, lithium will work in colder temperatures. Lithium batteries also have a much longer shelf life than alkaline batteries.

As for drawbacks, they are still not widely available. Alkaline batteries can be purchased in almost every supermarket, drug store, convenience store, and discount store in the United States. Lithium cells are much harder to find but are usually stocked by outdoors stores. Devices that use lithium cells require special bulbs, and there are restrictions about carrying them on aircraft. Under certain conditions (intense heat or prolonged shorting) lithium cells may explode, although it is more likely that they will release a small bit of sulfur-dioxide gas than explode. Lithium cells range in price from $8 for AA to $15 for a C to $20 for a D cell.

BEAR BAGS

A good deal of the Appalachian Trail wanders through bear country. Whether protected or hunted, bears love human food. A bear bag and a length of rope can be used to suspend a bag containing your food and other "smellables" from a tree to keep them out of reach of bears. Some shelters along the trail have bear boxes or other food storage arrangements but not all so you will want to have a rope available just in case.

ROPE

A length of rope, at least 25 feet long (and perhaps as long as 75 feet) approximately three-sixteenths of an inch in diameter, is absolutely necessary for hiking. Rope can be used for hanging your sleeping bags to air and hanging your wet clothes, rigging tents and tarps, lowering or pulling up a pack, hanging a pack from a tree, a belt, replacing frayed straps on gaiters or laces on boots, or for tying to a water bottle when it must be used as a dipper for water.

Keep in mind that if you intend to use a tarp on your backpacking trips you will probably need at least 50 feet of rope because you never know how far apart

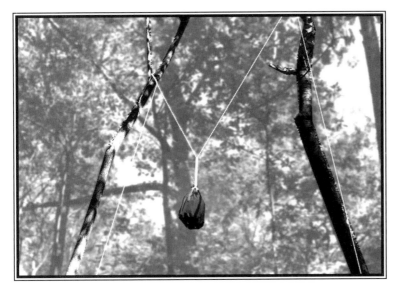

Food bag suspended from rope

the trees, rocks or shrubs will be that you will use to set it up. (Remember, too, that you can tie two lengths of rope together, if necessary.) Also, the tail of each knot should be at least a couple of inches long to insure that the knot won't slip.

Most outdoors stores offer several types of rope, but the best for general backpacking is heavy-duty twisted or braided nylon rope ranging in width from one-eighth of an inch to one-quarter of an inch (or three to eight millimeters). Before using nylon rope, always burn the ends into hard knobs so that the rope does not unravel.

TREKKING POLES

Many hikers, probably as many as 80 percent of thru-hikers, use one or even two trekking poles while hiking. They can provide physical benefits, taking stress off the knees and joints, and offering the opportunity to get upper body exercise. Older hikers with knee problems and hikers with injuries often say that they could not hike without them. Some tarps and ultralight tents use trekking poles as their tent poles, which allow you to get double use out of the high-tech hiking sticks.

However, there are some downsides from a minimum-impact perspective: trekking poles can gouge the treadway, hastening erosion and destroying the treadway built by volunteers. They also trample plants growing on the side of the trail, and leave scars on rocks unless rubber tips are used. Trekking poles are noisy, especially on rock. Rubber tips significantly reduce the noise but joints and springs can still make noise and be intrusive to other hikers.

Guns

Firearms are a controversial subject among hikers. Most hikers feel that guns are unnecessary, but a few do pack pistols or even rifles that will break down and fit into their packs.

Carrying weapons into a national park is a federal offense, and firearms are outlawed on other sections of trail as well. The real question is, are they necessary? To find out, we talked to hikers who, collectively, have hiked 80,000 miles on the A.T. as well as thousands of miles on the Pacific Crest, Continental Divide, and other trails, including some in Europe. We decided that if the hikers we talked to could walk that far without guns, we could prove a point. The bottom line was this: there was neither a single instance where a firearm was brought out of a pack (if one was carried), nor a case of a firearm helping a hiker out of a jam. None of the hikers we talked to, though some had carried guns, thought that firearms were necessary.

Guns do have a place, but the Appalachian Trail isn't one of them (unless, of course, it is hunting season; you have a license; and you are intentionally backpacking to a hunting spot). Animals, including humans, don't present enough danger to hikers to justify carrying firearms.

Cell Phones

Even more controversial than firearms, cell phones have become a flashpoint for hikers. Some hikers swear by the importance of having a cell phone to use in case of emergency. Other hikers swear at people who bring cell phones on a hike for an emergency only to phone a friend back home to describe the view from a mountain summit. Cell phones can provide an important link with search and rescue personnel or the police. However, cell phone service is spotty throughout the trail and a cell phone is certainly not essential. If you do decide to carry a cell phone, make sure that your phone does not ruin someone else's hike. Except in cases of emergency, never use your phone around other hikers. Turn off the ringer when sharing a shelter or tenting near others. Practice a little common courtesy and your phone will not be an issue for fellow hikers.

Your flashlight can do double duty as a lantern. Place an empty Nalgene bottle over the flashlight and stand the bottle up on the open end. The translucent bottle will diffuse the light and make a serviceable lantern.

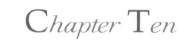

Chapter Ten

Potential Problems

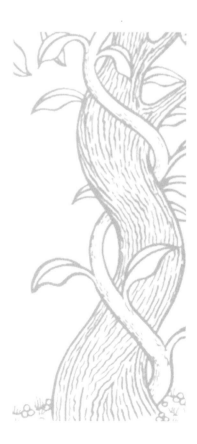

*Whenever you head out for a hike on the
Appalachian Trail, it is essential that
you are prepared. We have found that
preparation means planning. Make sure
that you have at least the bare minimum
of first aid along with you for a day hike
and a complete kit for longer hikes.
In thousands of miles of backpacking,
I have suffered only minor injuries that
were easily handled by a first-aid kit.
And it is unlikely you will have to deal
with anything more serious than a
scratch or two while on the trail. But
even the best-prepared hiker cannot
account for a seemingly unstable rock
that tips beneath the foot, twisted roots,
or even slippery pine needles.*

No one intends to hurt themselves when hiking. Victoria still bears the scar on her shin from a bad fall she took when she slipped on a wet rock. She had walked over hundreds of rocks that day. Why did that one throw her?

Whenever you head out for a hike on the A.T., it is essential that you are prepared. Being prepared for hiking is simply knowing what you are getting into and what to do when something unexpected happens—like running into a bear or spraining an ankle on a rock. Make sure that you have a basic first-aid kit along with you for a day hike and a more extensive kit for longer hikes. Because it is impossible to carry everything you might need for an outdoor emergency, your best bet is knowing how to improvise with what you have. You can carry a first-aid manual with you if you are really worried, but better to prepare by taking an appropriate first-aid or CPR class, or even a First Responder class (see Appendix Four, page 242). It doesn't do you any good to have a first-aid kit if you don't know how to use it.

Backpacking is more than just a walk in the woods. If you are not prepared to deal with the discomforts that are inherent in carrying a 30-plus-pound pack on your back, as well as the inconveniences involved in a backpacking trip, you should seriously reconsider getting into the sport. When backpacking, the outdoors is your home. You may have the shelter of a tent over your head at night, but other than that, the sky is your roof, and everything beneath it, including poisonous plants, nasty insects, rocks, roots, and mud, shares its home with you.

What follows are some of the possible "accidents" with which you might have to deal.

COLD-WEATHER AILMENTS

Hypothermia

Hypothermia is a killer and claims a number of lives each year, even in the middle of summer. The first signs of hypothermia—shivering, numbness, drowsiness, and marked muscular weakness—are followed by mental confusion and impairment of judgment, slurred speech, failing eyesight, and, eventually, unconsciousness.

Be aware of the most serious warning sign in an untreated hypothermia victim: when the shivering stops, the victim is close to death.

You are most likely to become hypothermic when you have stopped hiking, and especially if you are tired, which is likely if you have hiked more than a few miles that day. Movement keeps you warm, but when it is chilly outside and you are wet, your body's core temperature can drop once you become still.

Fortunately, hypothermia is easy to combat. If you arrive at your campsite or shelter on a cold, wet day and are experiencing any of the symptoms mentioned above, drop everything and make yourself warm. Strip yourself of your wet clothes and put on dry clothes, if possible. Crawl into your sleeping bag, and if you're able, heat something hot to drink—tea, soup, hot chocolate—anything hot will help raise your internal temperature. Drinks with a high sugar content are best. You may want to carry a pack of fruit gelatin. It tastes great when heated and contains a lot of sugar.

Once again, remember to take hypothermia seriously. Most hypothermia victims die in 40- to 50-degree weather.

FROSTBITE

Frostbite occurs when crystals begin to form either superficially or in the soft tissues of the skin. The effects of frostbite will be more severe if the affected area is thawed and then refrozen. Fortunately, the areas affected by frostbite are usually small. The nose, cheeks, ears, fingers, and toes are the most common areas.

Before frostbite occurs, the area will look flushed, then turning white or grayish yellow. Pain is often felt early but usually subsides—if you feel any pain at all.

If frostbite occurs, first cover the frozen area and provide the victim with extra clothing and blankets or double-wrap in sleeping bags. If possible, bring the victim indoors (a tent will do if nothing else is available) and provide him with a warm drink. Rewarm the frozen part quickly by immersing it in lukewarm water. Continue to keep the water warm. If warm water is not practical or available, wrap the affected part gently in warm blankets, clothes, etc.

Handle the frostbitten area gently. Do not massage it. Once thawed, the area will flush with blood and swell severely. At this point, discontinue warming it and have the victim exercise the part if possible. Severe pain will result as well.

Cleanse the frostbite area with water and soap and rinse it thoroughly before blotting it dry with clean towels or whatever you have handy that is clean and dry. If blisters have formed, do not break them.

If fingers or toes are involved, place gauze between them to keep them separated. Do not apply any other dressings unless you intend to transport the victim to medical aid. Also, elevate the frostbitten parts and protect them from contact with bedclothes. If toes are involved, the victim should not walk and additional heat should not be applied once the part is thawed. When you are alone and your feet and toes are frozen, do not attempt to thaw them out if you intend to walk to medical assistance.

If you decide to transport the victim, cover the affected areas with a clean cloth, apply temporary dressings, keep affected parts elevated, and continue to give victim fluids.

> *A note on windchill: When the wind starts to blow, even temperatures in the 50s can be dangerous. The lower the temperature and the greater the wind speed, the more hazardous the conditions. As I sit here writing this, an air temperature in the teens has the feel of below 0 degrees because of the 10-to-20-mile-per-hour winds.*

HOT-WEATHER AILMENTS

The three hot-weather ailments described below are serious problems and can be difficult to effectively treat on a hike. The best advice is to avoid problems by taking a few precautions in hot weather.

First, when you are hiking in the heat, try to maintain a consistent intake of fluids. Dehydration leads to these problems, so drinking lots of liquids will help avoid them. Second, if the heat starts to get to you, take a break. Sit down in the shade, drink some water, and give your body time to cool off.

HEAT CRAMPS

Heat cramps are an early sign of heat exhaustion, especially if the victim is dehydrated. Cramps occur first in the muscles of the legs and abdomen. If you're experiencing heat cramps, make a potassium solution:

METHOD 1: You will need two cups or water bottles. In one, mix eight ounces of potassium-rich fruit juice (apple, orange, or grapefruit) and add one teaspoon of honey or corn syrup (or sugar, if that is all you have available). Add a pinch of salt. In the other bottle, add eight ounces of a carbonated drink plus a quarter-teaspoon baking soda. Alternate sipping from each bottle until your thirst is quenched and both bottles are empty.

METHOD 2: Mix together one quart water, two tablespoons sugar, and a half-teaspoon salt. You could also add the half-teaspoon salt to a decaffeinated diet soda.

METHOD 3: To one quart of water, add two tablespoons sugar, a half-teaspoon Morton's lite salt, and an eighth-teaspoon table salt. For flavor, mix this concoction with diet Kool-Aid.

The key is to drink the solution slowly so that it can be absorbed by your body. If you drink it too fast, you may vomit, which adds even more stress to your body. Try drinking it over a period of an hour—sip, wait, sip, wait, an so on.

If you are going to be doing a lot of hiking in hot weather or are prone to overheating, you might want to carry along some Gatorade or similar drink or some potassium pills. Another option would be to make the sugar-and-salt solution, store it in a snack-size zipper-lock bag, and add it to your first-aid kit. Massaging will help relieve the cramped muscles.

HEAT EXHAUSTION

If heat cramps are not treated and lead to heat exhaustion, body temperature will be nearly normal. The victim's skin looks pale and feels cool and clammy. If the victim faints, lowering his head will help him regain consciousness. Weakness, nausea, and dizziness are, in addition to cramps, symptoms of heat exhaustion. As with heat cramps, the victim needs to drink an electrolyte solution as mentioned above. Lay the victim down, loosen his clothing, and raise his feet 8 to 12 inches above the level of the head. Applying cool wet cloths to the forehead, back of the neck, and armpits will also help relieve heat exhaustion.

Should the victim vomit, stop the solution intake. At this point, medical attention should be sought.

If you experience heat exhaustion on a hike, it would be wise to take a day off or even cancel the remainder of the hike.

HEAT STROKE

Treatment of heat stroke should be immediate. Cues include hot, red, and dry skin, a rapid pulse, and eventually unconsciousness.

Undress the hiker and bathe her skin with cool water or place her in a stream or other cold body of water if possible. Once her temperature lowers, dry her off. If cold water is not available, fan her with whatever you have on hand. If

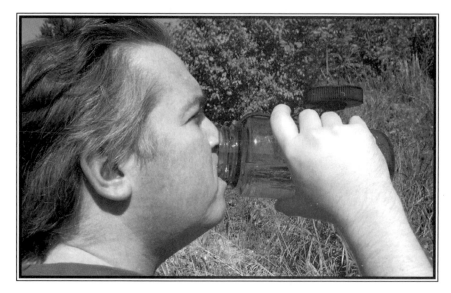

Staying hydrated on the trail is key to staying healthy.

her temperature rises again, resume the cooling process. Never give a hiker with heat stroke stimulants, such as tea.

Once the victim's temperature begins to drop, be careful not to overchill her. This can be as dangerous as the overheating she has just suffered. And, because the mortality rate associated with heat stroke is high, medical attention should be sought as soon as the hiker is stable enough to be moved.

Hyponatremia

Though some of us feel we can never drink enough water, especially when hiking in the middle of summer beneath a blazing sun, if you're not careful, you risk getting one of the lesser known heat illnesses.

Hyponatremia, also known as "water intoxication," is an abnormally low concentration of sodium in the blood. Sodium (salt and chloride) is an electrolyte, which helps the body distribute water. This is essential for water balance and for your muscles and organs to function effectively. Electrolytes are lost through sweat. When exercising, our body temperature rises and we sweat to keep cool. The more we sweat, the more sodium lost. The Gatorade Sports and Science Institute observes that sweat loss varies from as little as 16 ounces to over three quarts during each hour of exercise. It is vital that these body fluids are replaced both during and after exercise. To completely replace these fluids, you must replace not only water but also sodium and chloride.

Symptoms of hyponatremia include lightheadedness, nausea, vomiting, altered mental states, and frequent urination. Basically an imbalance of salt in your body (you have too little salt compared to the water in you), hyponatremia is treated by eating salty foods. Avoid relying solely on salt tablets, which may cause vomiting.

Long-distance hikers who take prescription medicine should consult a doctor, as some medications reduce the body's capability to conserve salt. Aspirin, ibuprofen, and other nonsteroidal anti-inflammatory agents interfere with kidney function and may also contribute to the development of hyponatremia in long-distance hikers.

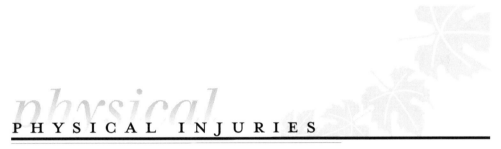

PHYSICAL INJURIES

BURNS

Cook pots are susceptible to tipping, and hikers are exposed to serious burns from the boiling contents as well as burns inflicted by the often-relentless summer sun. Sitting too close to a campfire and carelessly lighting your backpacking stove or igniting it in a tent are other ways to get burned.

First-degree burns appear bright red. Treat these minor burns by pouring cold water over the burned area and applying cold compresses for five to ten minutes. The skin should be allowed to air-dry if possible. Sunburn can be prevented by the use of a sunscreen with a sun protection factor of 30 or more. Continued exposure to sun can cause severe burns and may eventually lead to skin cancer. Antiseptic burn sprays may be used with first-degree burns.

Second-degree burns are characterized by bright-red skin, blisters, and swelling. Do not break the blisters if you plan to seek medical attention. Rather, immerse the burn in cold water or pour cold water over the burned area. Quick action will help reduce the burning effect of heat in the deeper layers of skin. Cover the burn with a sterile bandage. If you must hike on, a second-degree burn must be kept clean and will need to be treated with a triple-antibiotic ointment. Blisters that break should have the hanging skin removed. Ideally, a sterile piece of petrolatum gauze is placed over a generous application of ointment and then wrapped lightly

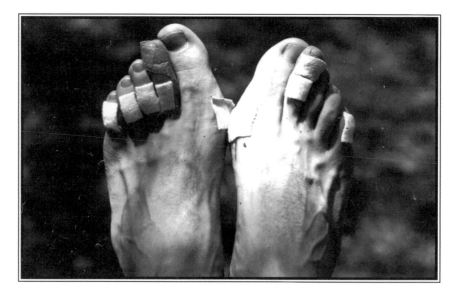

Be prepared to treat blisters—prevention, though, is best.

with sterile roll gauze. Change the bandage daily. After the burn stabilizes, a standard practice in burn units—and one that yields amazing results—is to swap out the triple-antibiotic for Preparation H. It sounds nutty, but a hemorrhoid cream such as Preparation H will dramatically speed the granulation of new tissue.

Third-degree burns are highly unlikely on a hike. These burns are distinguished by charred flesh and must be treated in a hospital. If third-degree burns occur, do not remove clothing, which may adhere to the burns. If you cannot get to a hospital within an hour, give the victim a potassium solution to sip on. Unlike first- and second-degree burns, do not immerse the burn in cold water. Cover the area with a clean cloth and get the victim to a doctor immediately.

BLISTERS

Blisters heal slowly, especially if you aggravate them by continuing to hike. The best way to avoid this problem is to treat blisters before they occur.

When a part of your foot feels hot or tender, stop hiking. Take your shoes and socks off and inspect the tender area. Cut out a piece of moleskin that is larger than the "hot spot" you will be covering. Apply the moleskin to the hot spot and put your socks and boots back on. Quick action at this stage may prevent blisters from developing. Duct tape may also be used to reduce the friction that leads to blisters; it comes in handy a lot of other ways. Wrapping a bit of duct tape around your water bottle is an easy way to have some on hand.

If you do get a blister, try to leave it unbroken. If it is still small and relatively flat, cover the blister with moleskin and resume hiking. Should the blister get worse, wash the area with soap and water, and then, with a sterilized needle (hold in a flame until the tip turns red; allow to cool a moment before using) make a small hole in the bottom of the blister so that the fluid drains. Once the blister is drained, apply a sterile bandage to prevent further irritation and infection.

If the blister is already broken, treat it like an open wound (cleanse and bandage it) and watch for signs of infection. If necessary, quit hiking for a day or two and let your blisters heal.

DROWNING

Knowing how to swim is essential for backcountry backpacking. You will often have to cross streams and on really hot days you will be tempted to immerse yourself in streams, ponds, and lakes even if you don't know how to swim. Between 6,000 and 8,000 people die each year by drowning. Drowning is a distinct possibility in the wilderness where caution is often thrown to the wind and certified lifeguards are nowhere to be found.

We have had two close calls while hiking—both times involved stream crossings after a storm. Once Victoria was nearly pulled beneath a log that she was using for support as she crossed a storm-swollen creek in Virginia. Another time Victoria was actually flipped over before she could grab a large boulder and keep herself from being swept downstream. Both times she was wearing a backpack.

It is essential to unfasten your hipbelt when packing across a stream, river, etc. Had she not been able to save herself at those moments, she would have been able to shrug off her pack and increase her chances for survival. A pack will drag you under and may be the deciding factor in whether or not you live or die.

If you come across someone who is drowning, remove the victim from the water if possible (but to be careful—don't create another drowning victim). If you can't remove him from the water, keep his head above water. Often foot entrapment or entanglement in a strainer, combined with a swift current, may make it extremely difficult to extract someone. Once the drowning victim has been removed from the water (and sometimes even before) you may have to perform artificial respiration. If there is no pulse, you will need to perform CPR. When dealing with a drowning, always send for help if possible. Without proper care a victim of near-drowning may contract lung infections and develop other problems that might lead to death.

Foot and Leg Problems

Extreme pain, and often swelling, characterizes hiking-related problems in the knees, shins, ankles, and feet. Taking a day or two off will often relieve the problem, but if the pain continues (or the swelling increases), only a doctor can tell you if your problem requires medical treatment.

It is not unusual for a hiker to experience some sort of pain every day he is on the trail. As one backpacker put it, "If the pain moves around, you're probably all right; but if it remains in one place, then it is more than likely something serious." Don't wait to see a doctor if there is swelling and continual pain. Nothing is worth causing permanent damage to your body. The doctor probably will prescribe an anti-inflammatory and tell you to keep off your feet for a week or more.

Even if you're hiking long distance, it's not the end of the world. Frank had shin splints while hiking the A.T. and was forced to take a week off. We still managed to complete the Trail in six months. But, had he not seen a doctor, he could have caused permanent damage to his calves.

One of the most common complaints is knee pain. Fortunately, the tenderness in the joints doesn't necessarily signal a problem. Aspirin or other pain relievers can help alleviate some of the pain. Wearing a knee brace can help prevent knee problems or aid in support once a problem develops. If you have a history of knee problems, it is a good idea to carry a brace just in case. If it is an emergency, try using a thick sock wrapped around your knee and bound with duct tape.

Also, keep in mind that if you have known problems with shin splints or other lower extremity problems, you can look into having orthotics made especially for your hiking boots. In most cases these can prevent shin splints.

Strains and Sprains

A strain is simply a stretched muscle (weightlifters stretch and actually tear muscle tissue to increase muscle bulk). A strained muscle should be treated with cold if the pain appears suddenly, with warmth if the pain sets in gradually. After a couple of days, heat should be used in most cases. The muscle can be used, but if it hurts don't do it.

A sprain, on the other hand, is a more serious injury. A sprain occurs when a joint and the ligaments that hold it are damaged. Unless treated properly, damage from a sprain can stay with you the rest of your life.

A sprain can be as simple as overstretching the ligament or as complex as tearing the ligament. Unfortunately, sprains don't hurt as much as they should and are often not treated until the awful swelling is noticed many hours later (and too late).

Treating a sprain is relatively simple, even in the backcountry. Take all pressure off the sprained body part immediately. Let's assume it's your ankle because that is the most likely thing you'll sprain while backpacking. Lie down and elevate your leg (that means make sure it's higher than your heart). Soaking a bandana or T-shirt in cold water can suffice as a cold compress—the evaporation will help cool the injury. Once numbed, let the injury re-warm for 10 to 15 minutes. Wrap an Ace (elastic) bandage (there should be one in your first-aid kit) around the sprained ankle. After applying a gauze pad over the swelling on the sprained joint, use "figure eight" winding to wrap the joint. Be careful not to wrap too tightly—you don't want to impair circulation.

Continue to use cold compresses on the injured joint for the next several days, and as soon as the swelling begins to recede, begin exercising the injured part. Never overdo it. If it starts to swell and ache again, retreat and begin the process over again. It is important that you exercise the sprain so that the muscles do not atrophy. And keep in mind that it will take a good two months before your joint is back to normal again.

FRACTURES

Fractures are serious injuries and will require evacuation from the backcountry. When someone has a possible fracture, your first move should be to look for swelling, discoloration, asymmetry, and severe pain. If you're not sure, assume it is a fracture.

Never try to set the fracture or straighten the injured part unless the limb is bent under the person and you are several hours from help. In that case, move the limb very gently. Wet clothing should be cut away so that the victim may be kept warm.

If the fracture is of the collarbone, upper arm, elbow, forearm, wrist, finger, ankle, or foot, you may be able to splint it. Use heavy sticks or tent poles for splints and bandanas or clothing for padding. Splinting should immobilize the joint above and below the injury unless the break is isolated in a joint. If the victim is able to walk, get him to help as soon as possible.

If the fracture is not in one of the places listed above, you should have the victim lie as quietly as possible. Protect and immobilize the injured area by surrounding it with sleeping bags, clothing, and other appropriate materials. Make sure the victim remains warm and go for help.

LIGHTNING

While playing Trivial Pursuit one night, our team was asked what natural phenomena claims the most victims each year. We thought about it—floods, earthquakes, tornadoes, tsunamis. We finally decided on floods because of the number of people killed during monsoon season. We fell out of our seats when we learned it was lightning. We hadn't even considered it. Really? Lightning?

Sure enough. Lightning kills between 100 and 300 people each year worldwide, particularly between May and September. An encyclopedia informed us that lightning strikes a hundred times a second worldwide, with each strike packing as much as 200 million volts, 300,000 amps, and 8,000 °C of heat. Ouch!

Lightning can strike three ways: within a cloud, cloud-to-cloud, and cloud-to-ground. Cloud-to-ground lightning can injure you in four different ways: by direct strike; by the splash or side flash, when lightning hits something else but flashes through the air to hit you as well; by ground current (the most common method of injuring humans), when the lightning strikes a tree, for instance, and the current runs through the ground or water and into you; and by the blast effect, when you are thrown by the sudden expansion of air caused by a strike. Some people get lucky when the ground current charge passes over and around them without entering their body. This is called the flashover effect.

There are a number of types of injuries a lightning victim can receive—traumatic, respiratory, neurologic, and cardiac injuries, as well as burns and everything from loss of hearing to vomiting. Treatment is for the type of injury the victim has sustained. Knowing CPR will be invaluable to you in a lightning case because most victims can be revived by this method. Never assume that a lightning-strike victim is fine. Always go for help.

According to the National Lightning Safety Institute, no one can predict where lightning will strike. Lightning can strike ten miles from an approaching thunderstorm. Once you see lightning flash or strike (or if you are more cautious, when you simply hear thunder), it's best to seek cover. Storms travel quickly and can be on you before you know it.

So what's safe? Not much. Avoid bodies of water and low places that can collect water. Avoid high places, open places, tall objects, metal objects, wet caves, and ditches. Your best bet is a small stand of trees. Sit on a sleeping pad (unless it has metal in it) with your knees pulled up against your chest, head bowed, arms hugging knees. If you're in a group, spread out but make sure you can all see at least one other person in case any one gets hit.

RASHES

The best thing to do once you realize you've been in contact with a plant prone to delivering rashes, such as poison ivy or nettles, is to take a cool or cold bath and completely cleanse yourself with soap. After that, use Calamine or a similar lotion. Cortisone creams help some (Victoria has had poison ivy so bad she needed cortisone shots). Antihistamines such as Benadryl (diphenhydramine) also offer some relief. Prophylactics are available, although how well they prevent rashes from poison plants is debatable.

Your best defense against poison ivy is to be able to identify and steer clear of it. As the saying goes—leaves of three, let them be.

Poison-ivy rash isn't the only rash you're likely to get while hiking. Rashes caused by friction, heat, and humidity are common, especially in the crotch area. One way to prevent rash is to apply Vaseline to any areas that rub against one another. If heat is the problem, try to keep the area as cool as possible. Shorts with built-in liners will keep you drier than shorts and underwear because they are made to allow moisture to escape. If the rash gets to be a real problem, try sleeping nude at night to allow the area to dry as thoroughly as possible. Powder will also help keep the problem area dry. If the rash becomes red and itchy, there are a number of over-the-counter products, such as Desenex, that will help clear it up.

Hip-belt rashes—when the hip belt is too loose and rubs the hiker's hips raw—are common. This happened to Victoria in the heat of the summer. The combination of the sweat and the hip

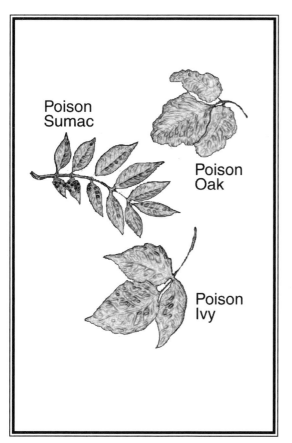

Poison ivy, oak, and sumac

belt rubbing through her cotton shorts soon caused a mean wound across her lower back in the shape of the hip belt. It bled and scabbed and bled and scabbed, and left her nearly frantic with pain. Changing to a pair of nylon shorts solved the problem—the material was slick enough to keep the hip belt gliding rather than rubbing against her hips. She already had the smallest hip belt available for the pack so getting a smaller one wasn't an option.

Another problem many hikers develop are swollen and bruised hips caused by the pressure of a heavy load on the hip belt. Other than lightening your pack, there is really no way to avoid this. Fortunately, every day you're on the trail the pack gets lighter until you resupply again. The welts on our hips usually disappeared a day or two after we settled an especially heavy load on our backs.

WOUNDS

It is not unusual to experience minor and sometimes major wounds—abrasions, incisions, lacerations, and punctures—while hiking. Avulsions, though rare, are also possible.

We still bear the scars of some of our falls, most of which involved slipping on leaves, roots, or rocks. Sometimes it doesn't matter how careful you are, you are just going to fall. Any backpacker can relate a major fall story. Our favorite is a fall that we wish we could have captured on video. It was really a very minor slope, but somehow Victoria slipped (on a rock or slick leaves) and her feet went flying out from under her. Soon she was rolling down the hill. Although Frank laughed, he soon found himself in the same predicament. It wasn't long before we were entangled and rolling down the slope together. It must have been a comic sight. Fortunately, neither of us suffered more than a few bruises to our bodies as well as our egos. We picked ourselves up, dusted off, and headed up the trail.

When someone is injured to such a degree that there is a flow of blood from the wound, you need to do three things: stop the bleeding, prevent infection, and promote healing.

Here are two methods, described in order of preference, that should be used to stop bleeding:

- With a dressing or a cloth, apply direct pressure over the wound. In most instances this will stop the bleeding, and the thick pad of cloth will absorb blood and allow it to clot. Once the blood clots, leave it alone. If blood should soak the pad before clotting, do not remove the pad but add another layer to the already soaked cloth and increase your pressure on the wound. If you need both your hands to help the victim, apply a pressure bandage with a strip of cloth. Place it over the pad on the wound, wrap it around the body part, and then tie a knot directly over the pad.

🖐 Unless there is evidence of a fracture, elevate the wounded part above the victim's heart. This will help reduce blood flow. Wounds of the hand, neck, arm, or leg should be elevated, and direct pressure should be continued.

These methods will stop most bleeding, but taking a course in first aid will teach you other options to use if the bleeding doesn't stop with direct pressure and elevation.

Preventing infection goes hand-in-hand with proper cleansing of the wound. Your first step is to wash your hands and to avoid contaminating the wound further. That is, don't breathe on it, cough or sneeze on it, drool on it, throw dirt on it, etc. Cleaning means cleansing around and sometimes in the wound. You can make an antiseptic wash by using the povidone-iodine in your first-aid kit or soap and water, or just plain water if that is all you have.

Cleanse around the wound with a sterile gauze pad, and in the wound if there is foreign material such as ground debris in it. Always rinse everything, even the antiseptic wash, from the wound before you dress it. You can irrigate the wound with water from a plastic bag that has a pin hole (to direct the stream of water).

If foreign matter remains in the wound after irrigation, you may try using sterilized tweezers to remove it (sterilize by holding them to a flame until red hot or by boiling them in water—make sure they cool down a bit before you apply them to the wound). If you can remove all foreign objects, and have stopped the bleeding, allow the wound to air-dry before dressing it. If you can't remove the debris, or the wound is too large to dress, keep it moist until you can get to a doctor. If it is a gaping laceration, cleanse the wound thoroughly and apply a butterfly bandage to pull the wound edges together. Some first-aid books do not advocate the use of butterfly bandages because it is felt that the bandages promote infection. Do as your conscience sees fit.

When dressing a wound, do not touch the sterile dressing except at the edges where it will not come in contact with the wound. If possible, the dressing should extend at least one inch past the edges of the wound.

The dressing should be bandaged snugly but not too tight. Remember to check it often, and never apply tape on the wound. Also, if you use tincture of benzoin on the healthy skin, the tape will stick better; don't get the benzoin in the wound because it will hurt and encourage infection.

ABRASIONS

Most of the wounds you'll suffer when hiking will be abrasions, which occur when the outer layers of the protective skin are damaged, usually when the skin is scraped against a hard surface.

Although bleeding is usually limited, danger of contamination and infection still exists. Simply cleansing the wound, applying an antiseptic, and keeping it clean until healed will avoid serious problems.

INCISIONS

An incision occurs when body tissue is cut with a sharp object. When hiking, most incisions are the product of poor knife handling. People can never seem to remember that they are supposed to cut away from their body. I've seen a number of hikers forced to head off for emergency help because they sliced their hands while whittling.

An incised wound often bleeds heavily and rapidly, and if deep, can damage muscles, tendons, and nerves. Incisions need immediate attention, even if small, because they can easily become infected. Whether a deep or shallow cut, the bleeding should be stopped immediately. If the wound is large, you should also treat for shock.

PUNCTURES

The most likely puncture wound you will receive while backpacking is a splinter. But if you walk around barefoot, you're asking for all manner of foot wounds. Keep shoes of some sort on at all times.

When several layers of skin are pierced by a sharp object, you have a puncture wound. Although bleeding is usually limited, internal damage can result if tissues and muscle are pierced. Infection is likelier because there is no flushing action from blood. Cleanse the wound; if there is a foreign object (such as a splinter) that is easily removable, remove it with a pair of sterilized tweezers or a needle. Objects imbedded deeply in the tissue should be removed only by a doctor.

AMPUTATION

If tissue is forcibly separated or torn from the victim's body, seek help as soon as possible. Bleeding will usually be heavy and should be stopped before transporting the victim, if possible. Send the avulsed body part along with the victim to the hospital. It can often be reattached.

GETTING HELP

getting help

T he above was a list of some of the more common emergencies you might face on a backpacking trip. There are a host of others—everything from abdominal pain to diabetic shock to spinal injuries. All of these take a knowledge of first aid that cannot be encompassed in this book. Taking a first-aid course will introduce you to these problems and teach you how to respond. See the appendix for contact information regarding first-aid related courses (page 242).

While talking to a couple of rangers, a friend of ours took a step backwards while saying farewell and stepped off a cliff. The rangers quickly sent for help, but it took a major evacuation effort before she could be reached and her injuries assessed. The two rangers, knowledgeable in wilderness first aid, were forced to make a judgment call on how to handle this outdoor emergency.

I can't tell you how to evacuate a person who has just fallen off a cliff, but if I had to make that decision, there are a number of questions I would have to consider. How far is help? Is the person still alive? Is there someone around more qualified to deal with the situation? Can the victim be reached? Is the temperature detrimental (too hot or too cold) to the victim? Is the victim breathing or bleeding? And so on.

In emergency situations that require evacuation you will be faced with many choices. But unless you are trained in wilderness rescue, you would be best advised to go for help rather than trying to evacuate the victim yourself. We can't put it more simply. Never evacuate the victim yourself. Let professionals handle it. If you try to evacuate the victim yourself, you may injure him or her further. And, unfortunately, that means you can be held liable.

Fortunately, most states have developed "Good Samaritan Laws." Most Good Samaritan Laws required that the person giving aid should not deliberately cause harm to the victim. The person giving aid also must provide the level and type of care expected of a responsible person with the same amount of training and similar circumstances. Finally, before one can give first aid, one must get permission from the injured party, unless that person is unconscious or unresponsive.

If a rescue and evacuation scenario develops, send for help as soon as possible. In the meantime, there are a number of things you can do to make the injured person more comfortable. According to *Emergency Medical Procedures for the Outdoors*, you can:

- ❧ Set up a shelter and protect the victim from direct contact with the ground if possible.
- ❧ Cover the victim with a shirt, jacket, sweater, etc., to retain body heat.
- ❧ Leave or provide food and water.
- ❧ Make sure victim is comfortable.

It's a dangerous world out there, and the Boy Scouts had the right idea when they chose as their motto the succinct "Be prepared." So, before you head out into the backcountry, be prepared. Or hike with someone who is.

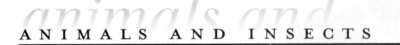

ANIMALS AND INSECTS

If you hike on the Appalachian Trail, you are bound to meet up with some sort of wildlife. Whether it be a lowly shelter mouse or the majestic moose, backpacking will give you a more intimate look at the animals you share the outdoors with. Sometimes people ask us if we have encountered problems with snakes and bears on the A.T. They want to hear a good story. What we tell them is that the only problem is not seeing them as often as we would like. After all, most every hiker–animal encounter is positive, a highlight of your hike.

Do not let the following words of caution discourage you from getting out on the Trail. The Trail belongs to the wildlife as well as the hikers, and a little caution and courtesy toward animals will go a long way. The following are among the animals that hikers are likely to meet while hiking on the A.T. You should know how to react to them to minimize potential problems.

BLACK BEARS

Black bears inhabit almost every region of the Appalachian Trail. They are usually shy, avoiding contact with humans. Hikers on most areas of the A.T. never see a bear. However, once a bear becomes habituated to people and learns to associate them with food, it may lose its fear of people. This can happen even in areas where bears are hunted. While black bears rarely inflict injuries, they can be aggressive in obtaining food.

Rangers in the Great Smoky Mountains National Park offer this advice: "If you see a bear at a distance, do no approach it. If your presence causes the bear to change its behavior (the bear stops feeding, changes travel direction, watches you, etc.) you are too close."

You will know if you are definitely too close when a bear reacts with aggressive behavior—swatting the ground, making loud noises, or charging at you. These behaviors show that the bear is demanding more space. Slowly back away, while maintaining a watchful eye on the bear. Do not run, but increase the distance between you and the bear slowly. In most every instance, the bear will do the same.

If the bear approaches or follows persistently, try changing your direction. If this does not work and the bear is still following, you will need to stand your ground. Shouting at the bear and acting aggressively should frighten it away. If you are with other hikers, work together to look as large as possible. Throw small rocks or other non-food objects at the bear. Use a deterrent such as a trekking pole, if you have one, or a stout stick if one is close at hand. Most importantly: do not run and do not turn away from the bear.

Do not leave food for the bear; this encourages further problems. Most injuries from black-bear attacks are minor and result from a bear attempting to get at people food. If the bear's behavior indicates that it is after your food and you are physically attacked, move yourself away from the food by slowly backing away.

If the bear shows no interest in your food and you are physically attacked, fight back aggressively with any available object. On the other hand, if it is a female black bear with cubs present, she will defend more aggressively and your best defense is to play dead.

Never, under any circumstances, try to feed a bear or leave food to attract them. Once a bear has tasted human food, he will continue to search for it, which means trouble for the bear as well as humans.

When making camp for the night, stash your food and all "smellables" in a bag and make sure it is securely tied off the ground and between two trees. The bag should be approximately 12 feet off the ground, 6 feet from the tree trunk, and 6 feet below the supporting limb.

In the areas that see the most bears—Georgia, the Nantahalas, the Smokies, Shenandoah National Park, and New Jersey—bearproof means of storage are provided for hikers. Food-storage devices include pully and cable systems, poles, and metal boxes.

SNAKES

In the wild, snakes lie in wait along a path for small rodents or other prey. Coiled along the edge of a trail, waiting for food to pass by, the patient reptiles test the air with their flicking tongues for signs of game.

This image of the snake lying in wait just off the trail is a cause of concern among some hikers; but what about the snake's view of things? The snake is aware of its place in the food chain; it must watch for predators as well as prey. A hiker making a moderate amount of noise will usually be perceived as a predator and the snake will back off or lie still until the "danger" passes.

Garter snakes, ribbon snakes, and black rat snakes are among the non-venomous snakes commonly found in the Appalachian mountains. Rattlesnakes and copperheads are the only species of venomous snake you could possibly encounter on the Appalachian Trail. Both the rattlesnake and copperhead are not aggressive and will avoid striking a human unless cornered.

To avoid confrontations with snakes, remember to make a little extra noise when you are walking through brush, deep grass, or piles of dead leaves that block your view of the footpath. Though the snakes cannot hear the noise, they do sense the vibrations, which warn them of your approach. By kicking at the brush or leaves slightly, you will make enough noise to cause a snake to slither off or lie still.

The sad truth is that the majority of snakebites occur on and around the hand. This is because folks pick up the snake, venomous or otherwise, for a closer look. Ankle and leg bites are very rare.

Both species of venomous snake prefer areas near rocky outcrops, and copperheads can be found among the boulders that border rocky streams as well. Viewpoints, such as Zeager Cliffs in Pennsylvania, are popular sunning spots for snakes. Venomous snakes do not occur as far north as Maine, and copperheads do not commonly appear in Vermont and New Hampshire. Here are some tips for recognizing these two venomous snakes.

COPPERHEADS

Copperheads are typically two to three feet in length. They have moderately stout-bodies with brown or chestnut hourglass-shaped crossbands. The background color is lighter than the crossbands, anything from reddish brown to chestnut to gray-brown. The margins of the crossbands have a darker outline. This pattern certainly helps the copperhead blend in among dead leaves. Similarly marked but nonvenomous snakes (e.g., corn snake) have similar markings, but none are so distinctively hourglass-shaped.

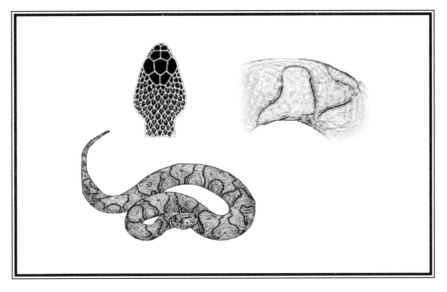

Copperhead

Copperheads prefer companionship; if you see one copperhead, there are probably other in the area. In the spring and fall they can be seen in groups, particularly in rocky areas.

Copperheads avoid trouble by lying still and will quickly retreat as a last resort. The bite of a copperhead is almost never fatal. Rarely has someone weighing more than 40 pounds died of a copperhead bite. The bite produces discoloration, massive swelling, and severe pain. While not fatal, the bite is dangerous and medical attention should be sought immediately.

RATTLESNAKES

Rattlesnakes are heavy-bodied and can be anywhere from three to five feet long, though large rattlesnakes are increasingly rare. Rattlesnakes also have dark blotches and crossbands (though these are not hourglass-shaped). There are two color phases (i.e., the background color)—a yellowish phase and a dark, almost black one. Sometimes their overall color is dark enough to obscure the pattern. A real giveaway is the prominent rattle or enlarged "button" on the end of the tail. Rattlesnakes usually warn predators with a distinctive rattle; but this can't be relied on because they may also lie still while hikers go by.

Because of the rattlesnake's size and resulting larger store of venom, its bite is more serious than that of the copperhead. But like the copperhead, it will strike only as a last resort.

Rattlesnakes are frequently seen on the Trail, though their presence has been greatly reduced by development encroaching on their terrain. Cases of

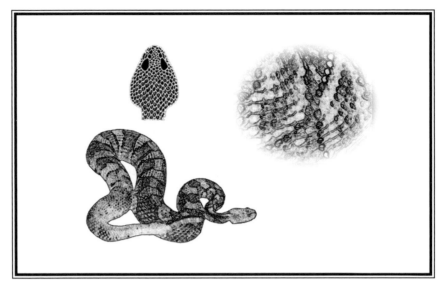

Rattlesnake

rattlesnake bites are almost unheard of, and when quick action is taken they will almost never prove fatal, except among the very young or very old.

TREATING NONVENOMOUS SNAKEBITES

By making a little extra noise in areas where snakes may be hidden from view, you should avoid any chance of a snakebite. If a bite should occur, proper treatment is important.

    If not properly cleaned, the wound can become infected. Ideally, the victim should be treated with a tetanus shot to prevent serious infection. Nonvenomous snakebites will cause a moderate amount of swelling. If large amounts of swelling take place, the bite should be treated as if it were caused by a venomous snake.

TREATING VENOMOUS SNAKEBITES

While a venomous snakebite on the A.T. is extremely rare, it is possible, particularly if you venture off the Trail and into the snake's habitat. Both rattlesnake and copperhead venoms are hemotoxins, which destroy red blood cells and prevent proper blood clotting. Organ degeneration and tissue damage result from the venom. Hemotoxins are quite painful and may result in permanent damage, so swift treatment is essential. Discoloration and swelling of the bite area are the most visible signs. Weakness and rapid pulse are other symptoms. Nausea, vomiting, fading vision, and shock also are possible signs of a venomous bite and may develop in the first hour or so after being bitten.

The best treatment is to reduce the amount of circulation in the area where the bite occurred and seek medical attention immediately. Circulation can be reduced by keeping the victim immobile (which isn't easy if the bite occurs five miles from the nearest road); by applying a cold, wet cloth to the area; or by using a constricting band. A constricting band is not a tourniquet and should be tight enough only to stop surface flow of blood and decrease the flow of lymph from the wound. The constricting band should not stop blood flow to the limb.

Tourniquets can cause more damage to the victim than a snakebite. If improperly applied, the tourniquet can cause the death of the infected limb and the need for amputation. The cutting and suction methods called for in snakebite kits also are not recommended.

BOAR, MOOSE, AND OTHERS

Boars, which are not indigenous to the United States (they were brought here from Europe for hunting purposes), can be found in the southern Appalachians, especially in the Great Smoky Mountains National Park. They are rarely seen and, like most animals, will disappear if they hear you coming. Should you happen upon a boar, try to avoid direct confrontation; just continue hiking.

Male moose should be avoided during rutting season because they may mistake you for a rival and attempt to chase you out of their territory.

Females of any and all species should be avoided when they have their young with them. The instinct for protecting their young is strong and you cannot predict what a mother will do if she feels her children are threatened.

Birds are especially vicious, but generally harmless. You may not see the grouse and her babies but she'll spot you and let you know that she is not pleased with your presence.

Only the very lucky will catch glimpses of other wild animals—wild cats, wolves, coyotes. Chances of confrontation are slim but, if you do, admire the view and keep walking.

SHELTER PESTS

Appalachian Trail shelters attract rodents and other small mammals. These creatures are searching for food and can do much damage, especially if you do not take care to protect your belongings.

It is never wise, even when camping along the A.T., to leave your pack, and particularly your food, out on the ground or shelter floor for the night. Food, and sometimes whole packs, should be hung where these animals cannot reach them.

PORCUPINES

These nocturnal creatures are shelter pests in the New England states. They love to gnaw on outhouses and shelters and are particularly fond of hiking boots and backpack shoulder straps. That may sound strange, but they are after the salt from your sweat. So hang your packs and boots when you're hiking in New England, and take particular care in shelters that are known to be frequented by porcupines. Fortunately, most of the shelters have been porcupine proofed: metal strips have been placed along the edges of the shelters to prevent the rodents from chewing on it.

Direct contact is necessary to receive the brunt of the porcupine's quills. Although it is unlikely for a hiker to be lashed by a porcupine's tail, it is not unusual for a dog to provoke a porcupine into defending itself. If your dog is attacked and you see quills, you either must pull them with pliers yourself or (preferably) seek help from a veterinarian.

Porcupine quills become embedded in the flesh of the attacker, causing extreme pain. If the quills are not removed immediately, they can cause death, as the quills will continue to work their way through the body in a straight line from the point of entry.

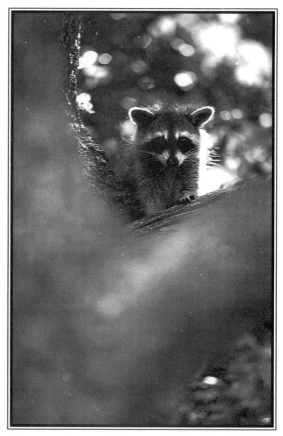

Raccoon

SKUNKS

Skunks inhabit the entire length of the Trail but are really only a problem for hikers in the Smokies. Dogs, on the other hand, can provoke skunk attacks from Georgia to Maine. Although we saw skunks only in the Smokies, we were aware of their presence (that telltale odor!) our entire trip.

During a night at Ice Water Springs Shelter north of Newfound Gap in the Smokies, a brazen skunk wove around our legs as we warmed ourselves in front of the campfire. It was very pleasant, scrounging for scraps of food on the shelter's dirt floor and along the wire bunks. The skunk occasionally stood on its hind legs and made a begging motion, which had no doubt been perfected on earlier hikers. We didn't give in to the skunk's pleas for food, and it eventually crawled back up under the bunks as we sighed in relief.

We heard of another skunk encounter in the same shelter, perhaps with the same skunk, a year earlier, when two British hikers, who were unfamiliar with the animal, tried to chase the skunk away by throwing a boot. They were given a quick course in skunk etiquette!

MICE

Mice are the most common pests in shelters. It doesn't take long after a new shelter has been built for the mice to arrive. The Appalachian Trail Conservancy states that the shelters are not the place to store, cook, or eat food. Not only will this keep mice out of shelters, but it will reduce other problems. One example is instructive.

In the 1990s, tuna cans suspended on rope started to appear in front of shelters along the Trail. These clever devices were intended to serve as "mouse baffles," a barrier to mice climbing down onto food bags. Whether the tuna cans discouraged mice or not, the ropes encouraged hikers to hang their smellable bags in the shelters. Bears soon came to see these as meals on a rope.

If you leave your pack sitting on the floor of a shelter, plan on the mice gnawing their way into your pack chasing smells and helping themselves to a mouse-sized portion of your gear. While we were hiking in Virginia, Victoria decided to change into a warmer shirt mid-morning, and was shocked to find that mice had gnawed several holes in the shirt's collar.

HANTAVIRUS

This virus was first identified during the Korean War and it was named for the Hantaan River there. An abundant crop of pinon nuts in the Southwest in 1993 led to an increased mouse population which in turn led to that area of the country being the first to experience widespread hantavirus. Unfortunately, the deadly strain of the virus that has developed in the United States occurs in backcountry areas, making it a concern for backpackers.

Hantavirus causes a respiratory disease that is carried in wild rodents such as deer mice. People become infected after breathing airborne particles of urine or saliva. Most cases have been associated with 1) occupying rodent-infested areas while hiking or camping; 2) cleaning barns or other outbuildings; 3) disturbing rodent-infested areas while hiking; 4) harvesting fields; or 5) living in or visiting areas that have experienced an increase in rodents.

The virus produces flu-like symptoms and takes one to five weeks to incubate. It has been fatal in 60 percent of victims.

PROBLEM INSECTS

You can't escape them. They're everywhere. Even in the coldest reaches of the Arctic and Antarctic, it is not surprising to stumble upon a bug. Mosquitoes, bees, hornets, wasps, fire ants, scorpions, ticks, chiggers, black flies, deer, and horse flies, gnats and no-see-ums are among the millions of insects out there that torment the human soul. . . and skin.

They invade our lives both indoors and out and, to be perfectly honest, we find insects much easier to deal with in the out-of-doors than inside our home or car. They may be demons outside, but they are Satan incarnate when trapped somewhere they do not want to be. So because you can't live with them and you can't live without them, how do you handle insects, especially those that sting, bite, and enjoy feasting on human blood?

BEES, HORNETS, WASPS, YELLOW JACKETS

We've only experienced one yellow jacket sting in thousands of miles of hiking. Mostly, these insects will try to avoid you but they are attracted to food, beverages, perfume, scented soaps, and lotions (including deodorant) and bright-colored clothing. Also, they nest anywhere that provides cover—in logs, trees, even underground.

Yellow jackets are the most obnoxious of the bunch, often stinging more than once and without provocation. By keeping your camp clean and food and drink under cover, you should avoid these stinging pests.

If stung by one of these insects, wash the area with soap and water to keep the sting from becoming infected. Apply a cool cloth for about 20 minutes to reduce swelling, and take an oral antihistamine such as Benadryl (diphenhydramine) to reduce swelling as well.

Check your damp clothing and towels before using to make sure a stinging insect has not alighted on it. And remember, bees, hornets, and wasps kill more people in the United States each year than snakes do.

Numerous stings can induce anaphylactic shock, which can be fatal. Those who know they are allergic to bee stings should carry an Anakit (available by prescription) with them into the backcountry. The kit contains a couple of injections of epinephrine and antihistamine tablets. Your doctor should be able to prescribe one for you. If you must use the injection, always get to a hospital as soon as possible for follow-up care.

Anaphylactic shock occurs when the body produces too much histamine in reaction to a bite or sting. The reaction turns your skin red, itchy hives appear, and airways begin to close down, sometimes completely, causing asphyxiation.

If you are presented with a case of anaphylaxis, give the victim antihistamine tablets if they can swallow, or inject epinephrine (follow kit directions) if available. You should be carrying Benadryl or some similar antihistamine in your first-aid kit. Seek help immediately.

For those not allergic to bites and stings, Sting-eze is supposed to be a superior product when it comes to relieving the pain and itching caused by most insects. It is said to combat infection from poison oak, cuts, burns, and abrasions.

BLACKFLIES, DEERFLIES, HORSEFLIES

Most abundant during late spring and summer, these flies produce a painful bite and leave a nasty mark on your skin. They sponge up the blood produced by their bite, which is why the wound is often so big. Deerflies, in particular, seem to prefer to dine on your head. When swarmed by the monsters, I have wrapped my head in two bandanas to avoid their bites. If bitten, wash with soap and water and use an oral antihistamine to reduce swelling and itching.

MOSQUITOES

When camping, there is nothing worse than a mosquito caught in your tent with you. They always seem to vanish, mysteriously, when you turn your flashlight on. Only the females bite (the males like the nectar found in flowers), but there always seem to be plenty of them around.

With cases of West Nile virus becoming increasingly common, mosquitoes are more than a minor nuisance. According to the Centers for Disease Control and Prevention, only 1 in 150 people who come in contact with the virus will develop a severe case of the illness. People typically develop symptoms between 3 and 14 days after they are bitten by the infected mosquito.

Progressive symptoms include high fever, headache, neck stiffness, stupor, disorientation, coma, tremors, convulsions, muscle weakness, vision loss, numbness, and paralysis. These symptoms may last several weeks, and neurological effects may be permanent. However, about 80 percent of people infected with

West Nile virus will show no symptoms at all. You are more likely to manifest symptoms of the virus if you are over 50 years of age.

Most of the time it is impossible to avoid mosquitoes, but if you camp in open, breezy areas away from still water, there's a good chance your sleep will be mosquito-free. Go for light-colored clothing that is too thick for mosquitoes to penetrate. If they are really thick, wear long-sleeved shirts and pants and use DEET, which is applied to your clothing rather than your skin.

Wash mosquito bites and use an oral antihistamine to reduce swelling. A paste of baking soda and water also often helps reduce the itching of mosquito bites.

SPIDERS

Anyone who has walked on the A.T. in the early morning has wiped spider webs off his or her face. While most spiders are harmless, there are some poisonous ones. Although it is a fairly unusual occurrence, a few hikers have had unpleasant encounters with brown recluse spiders. The initial bite may not even be felt, but pain will develop within several hours, along with symptoms that may include fever, chills, sweating, nausea, general malaise, and itching around the site. The main sign of this poisonous spider's bite is a bulls-eye rash, with a dark red or blue center, ringed with red, with another ring of white around it. If you develop these symptoms, seek immediate medical help. Treatment should be received within 48 hours to avoid possible tissue loss. While coma and death can occur, particularly in small children, that is very rare.

Be sure to shake out your clothing and boots before putting them on in the morning.

TICKS

A relative of spiders (another insect that leaves nasty bites), the tick has become a serious health threat. It is the carrier of both Rocky Mountain Spotted Fever and Lyme disease. Rocky Mountain Spotted Fever is carried by the wood ticks (west), lone star ticks (southwest), and dog ticks (east and south). Lyme disease is carried by the deer tick, which is about the size of a pinhead.

Whenever you are hiking in tick country—tall grass and underbrush—make sure you check yourself for ticks at the end of each day or more often if you actually notice one on your clothing while hiking. Wearing a hat, long-sleeved shirt, and pants with cuffs tucked into socks will also discourage ticks. This can be very uncomfortable in hot weather. Using a repellent containing permethrin will also help, as will keeping to the center of the trail.

Like mosquitoes, ticks are attracted to heat, often hanging around for months at a time waiting for a hot body to pass. Wearing light-colored clothing will allow you to see ticks. If a tick attaches itself to your body, the best way to remove it is to grasp tick with tweezers and pull, then wash the bite area. Once removed, carefully wash the bite with soap and water.

It takes a while for a tick to become imbedded. If you check yourself thoroughly after each hike—every mole and speck of dirt as well—you are more likely to catch the tick before it catches you. Tick season lasts from April through October, and peak season is from May through July. But in the South, tick season may last year-round if there has been a warmer-than-average winter.

Lyme Disease

More than 23,763 cases of Lyme disease were reported in 2002. The A.T. runs through prime Lyme-disease territory. Ninety-five percent of all cases of Lyme disease come occur in 12 states, 8 of which—Connecticut, Maine, Maryland, Massachusetts, New Jersey, New Hampshire, New York, and Pennsylvania—are also Trail states.

Among the symptoms of Lyme disease are fever, headache, pain, and stiffness in joints and muscles. If left untreated, Lyme disease can produce lifelong impairment of muscular and nervous systems, chronic arthritis, brain injury, and in ten percent of victims, crippling arthritis.

Lyme disease proceeds in three stages (although all three do not necessarily occur):

The first stage may consist of flu-like symptoms (fatigue, headache, muscle and joint pain, swollen glands) and a skin rash with a bright red border. Antibiotic treatment wipes out the infection at this stage.

The second stage may include paralysis of the facial muscles, heart palpitations, light-headedness, shortness of breath, severe headaches, encephalitis, and even meningitis. Other symptoms include irritability, stiff neck, and difficulty concentrating. Pain may move around from joint to joint.

The third stage may take several years to occur and consists of chronic arthritis with numbness, tingling and burning pain, and may include inflammation of the brain itself. The disease can also lead to serious heart complications and attack the liver, eyes, kidney, spleen, and lungs. Memory loss and lack of concentration are also present.

Although antibiotics are used for treatment in each stage, early detection and diagnosis are critical. If you suspect you have Lyme disease, see a doctor immediately.

REPELLENTS

DEET is the hands-down winner when it comes to repelling insects. Short for N-diethyl-meta-toluamide, DEET is found in some percentage in most repellents—lotions, creams, sticks, pump sprays, and aerosols.

This colorless, oily, slightly smelly ingredient is good against mosquitoes, no-see-ums (midges), fleas, ticks, gnats, and flies. Although it can range in percentage from 5 to 95 percent, the most common formulations contain approximately 35 percent DEET.

Repellents containing DEET in the 35-percent range are (in ascending order): Deep Woods Off! lotion, Deep Woods Off! towelettes, Cutter's Stick, Cutter's Cream, Cutter's Cream Evergreen Scent, Cutter's Cream Single Use Packets (35 percent), Muskol Ultra Maximum Strength, Repel, and Kampers Lotion (47.5 percent, and includes suntan lotion).

The Centers for Disease Control and Prevention notes that permethrin (which kills ticks on contact) may also be used, but it must be applied to clothes only and not to skin.

Avon's Skin-So-Soft is a highly recommended deterrent against no-see-ums and some bigger bugs such as sand fleas and black flies. It appears to work differently on each person. Victoria has had better luck with it than Frank has, for example.

DOGS

Some dogs encountered on the trail are hiking companions and others are strays or property of people who live along the Trail's route. They can be very friendly as well as hard to get rid of when they are strays. They can also be aggressive, especially if they feel they are defending their territory or their masters.

Fortunately, most of the dogs you meet on the A.T. are friendly. While hiking over The Humps (Tennessee) in the aftermath of a snowstorm, we were forced to contend with high winds and limited visibility as well as snow that ranged in depth from two inches to three-foot drifts. A stray dog had appeared at the shelter the previous night, and joined us when we set out for the eight-mile trip to town that morning.

As we climbed blindly over the wind-blown balds, the dog unerringly led us along the Appalachian Trail. At one point, a road very clearly led straight ahead while the Trail turned off to the left. We did not notice the Trail's turning, but the dog did. He turned left and we followed. Soon we saw blazes at the edge of the woods. Several times during that eight-hour hike, the dog kept us from wandering off the Trail and into the woods when the Trail's white-blazed trees were hidden beneath snow that had stuck to the trunks.

We also had bad experiences with dogs. In Vermont, a huge Newfoundland stood on its hind legs, barely two inches from Victoria's face, and growled, menacingly, his teeth bared. The tactic was apparently a very frightening bluff, which left us (and many other hikers) shaking. Stories of this particular dog filled the register at the next shelter.

HOW TO AVOID TROUBLESOME DOGS

As with bears and most other animals, don't run. Don't look directly into a dog's eyes, but if it is necessary to defend yourself, use your hiking stick or small stones. Sometimes just picking up a stone and holding it as if you're going to throw it is enough to dissuade a dog. Throw the rock only if it's absolutely necessary.

DOGS AS HIKING PARTNERS

Although dogs can make wonderful hiking partners, most hikers say they really prefer not to hike around people who are hiking with dogs. Unless you have complete control over your animal, you are probably going to make a lot of people unhappy, especially if you intend to stay in a shelter. Two of the biggest complaints from hikers were about wet dogs climbing all over their sleeping bags and other gear, and dogs who tried to eat their food.

If you plan to take a dog, remember that dogs usually are not welcomed by other hikers and do not have priority when it comes to shelter space. Dogs also are not allowed in the Great Smoky Mountains National Park (Tennessee and North Carolina), Trailside Museum and Wildlife Center in Bear Mountain State Park in New York, or in Baxter State Park in Maine. At Bear Mountain, there is an alternate road walk for hikers with dogs. On lands under the administration of the National Park Service (NPS), dogs are required to be on a leash. Approximately 40 percent of the Trail—lands acquired specifically to protect the A.T. (about 600 miles) and five of the six other units of the national park system that the Trail crosses: The Blue Ridge Parkway, Shenandoah National Park, the Harpers Ferry and C&O Canal national historic parks, and the Delaware Gap National Recreation Area—are covered by this rule. Dogs are also required to be on a leash through most of Maryland.

Dogs also tend to scare up troublesome run-ins with porcupines and snakes, for example. People hiking with dogs should be aware of the impact of their animals on the Trail environment and their effect on the Trail experience of others:

- Do not allow your pet to chase wildlife.

- Leash your dog around water sources and in sensitive alpine areas.

- Do not allow your dog to stand in springs or other sources of drinking water.

- Be mindful of the rights of other hikers not to be bothered by even a friendly dog.

- Bury your pet's waste as you would your own.

- Take special measures at shelters. Leash your dog in the shelter area, and ask permission of other hikers before allowing your dog in a shelter. Be prepared to "tent out" when a shelter is crowded, and on rainy days.

Also, if you choose to hike with a dog, you probably won't see much wildlife. If you wish to backpack or hike with your dog along the Appalachian Trail, you will probably want to read "Hiking with Fido," an article by veterinarian Tom Grenell. The article is available through the ATC or can be downloaded from their Web site, **www.appalachiantrail.org.**

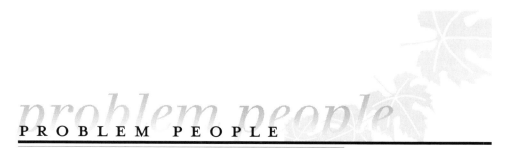

PROBLEM PEOPLE

In 1990 the murders of Geoff Hood and Molly LaRue in a Pennsylvania shelter sent shock waves through the hiking community. Even the nation felt the impact of their untimely and violent deaths as national news picked up the story. How could something like that happen in the wilderness?

Unfortunately, this is not the first time such a tragedy has occurred on the Appalachian Trail. It is doubtful it will be the last. Although in its 50-plus-year history the A.T. has seen only seven murders, it's location along the highly populated east coast makes it prone to problems involving humans. Rapes, thefts, and general harassment are also reported.

Why? Because where there are humans there are problems. Your safety, on the Appalachian or any trail, cannot be guaranteed. But following these guidelines will help:

DON'T HIKE ALONE. If you are by yourself and encounter a stranger who makes you feel uncomfortable, say you are with a group that is behind you. Be creative. If in doubt, move on.

LEAVE A TRIP ITINERARY AND TIMETABLE. Someone at home should know this information. Be sure they know your "trail name," if you use one. Check in regularly, and establish a procedure to follow if you fail to check in.

BE WARY OF STRANGERS. Be friendly, but cautious. Don't tell strangers your plans. Avoid people who act suspiciously, are hostile, or intoxicated. The Trail is known for the generosity bestowed upon hikers by townspeople or "trail angels" along the way, but think twice before accepting an offer that may potentially compromise your safety.

DO NOT CAMP NEAR ROAD CROSSINGS.

DRESS CONSERVATIVELY. Flamboyant or overly revealing clothing may attract unwelcome attention.

DON'T CARRY FIREARMS. Without a permit they are illegal on National Park Service lands and in most other areas. They could also be turned against you; you face a risk of an accidental shooting; and they add extra weight. The ATC strongly discourages the carrying of firearms.

ELIMINATE OPPORTUNITIES FOR THEFT. Do not bring jewelry. Hide your money. Do not leave your pack unattended in towns or close to road crossings. Don't leave valuables or equipment (especially in sight) in vehicles parked at road crossings. (Check the ATC Web site for current information on parking areas with known vandalism problems.)

USE TRAIL AND SHELTER REGISTERS. Sign in, leave a note, and report any suspicious activities. If someone needs to locate you, or if a serious crime has been committed along the Trail, the first place authorities will look is in the registers. Make sure your family knows your trail name if you use one.

REPORT ANY CRIME OR HARASSMENT. Notify local law-enforcement authorities and the ATC. You can download an online incident report form at the ATC Web site, contact the ATC at (304) 535-6331, or e-mail them at incident@ appalachiantrail.org. Report all occurrences of vandalism to both local authorities and the ATC, so that the Conservancy can pass along reports of problems to other hikers.

HUNTING

U p until 2002, no hunting accidents had ever been reported along the Trail. Then in the fall and winter of 2002–2003, two hikers were accidentally shot and seriously injured by hunters. One victim was a newbie backpacker relieving herself in the morning, the other an experienced long-distance hiker on a daily walk near his home. Both hikers were mistaken for deer; neither was wearing blaze orange. Both hunters were, of course, grossly negligent in following the basic practice of positively identifying their target, yet they were in National Forests where hunting is permitted.

Hunting is allowed on at least some portion of the Trail in every state the A.T. passes through. This includes national forests, state game lands, some state forests and other types of lands. Even on the National Park Service corridor lands, where hunting is prohibited, hunters may wander over from adjacent lands, which allow hunting without realizing they have crossed over onto federal lands.

The following precautions will help ensure your safety when hiking during hunting season:

UNDERSTAND LOCAL REGULATIONS: Call the state fish-and-game office to find out when and where hunting is allowed in the areas you intend to hike. A state-by-state overview is found at ATC's Web site, **www.appalachiantrail.org.**

WEAR BLAZE ORANGE: When hiking in fall, winter and spring, blaze orange will keep you from looking like a target. The blaze orange must be visible from both the front and back. Not only is it a good idea to wear blaze orange, it is required in Pennsylvania Game Lands, through which the Trail passes. From November 15 to December 15, except on Sundays, all persons on the state game lands must wear at least 250 square inches of fluorescent orange.

BE HEARD: Make sure you are heard by hunters by whistling, singing or talking. Any noise which is unambiguously human will be helpful.

USE CAUTION NEAR ROADS AND IN VALLEYS: Be especially cautious when within a half mile of road crossings.

AVOID DEER FIREARM SEASON: Of course, the safest option is to stay off portions of the Trail where hunting is allowed during deer firearm season.

Chapter Eleven

Preparing for Your First Hike

Here's the best advice when it comes to your first hike: Don't bite off more than you can chew. When starting out, it is very easy to run yourself into the ground, and it takes a lot longer to hike ten rugged miles than you think.

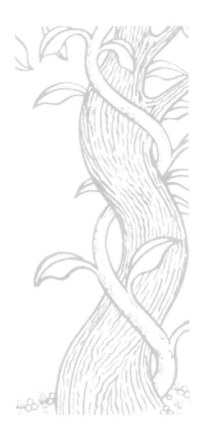

HOW FAR AND HOW FAST?

P hil Hall had a novel idea for training for his first hike: "I carried around a 70-pound bag of birdseed on my shoulders for ten miles over a ten-day period," he said. "From this, I got a tired and sore neck but discovered a clever way of easily hitching rides."

Phil realized the folly of his plan, chucked the bag of birdseed, and took the direct approach.

"I then decided that I would just start out slowly and do however many miles I could."

He had the right idea. The only way to adjust to backpacking is to backpack. Unfortunately, there is no other way to prepare. Being in good cardiovascular condition helps, but you don't have to be in great shape to backpack. Whether you're in good shape or not, you should allow yourself time to adjust.

So how far should you hike? When you first start hiking, don't plan on more than ten miles a day. A five-mile day hike is an even better choice. This will give you plenty of time to enjoy the scenery without overextending yourself. For an overnight "shakedown" hike, you may want to keep the mileage about the same, certainly no more than 15 miles over two days. This will allow you to test how well you prepared and packed without overextending yourself. After several shorter hikes, you may decide that you can extend your backpacking trips without ruining the fun.

Once you are on the trail, don't count on more than a one-mile-per-hour pace with a full pack. For a five-mile hike, allow yourself five hours. Your actual walking pace will probably be faster, but your body will crave frequent breaks. A lot of people assume that a four-mile-an-hour pace is standard. Well, it is if you're walking around a track or on a level stretch of road without a pack. But even the most seasoned hiker finds it next to impossible to keep a four-mile-an-hour pace on tough terrain. A one-and-a-half-to-two-mile-per-hour pace is average for a hiker in peak condition.

It won't take long before you begin approaching a two-mile-per-hour pace. As you get experience, a good rule of thumb for planning your trip is to allow an hour for every two miles of trail plus one hour for each 1,000 feet of elevation to be gained. So, for a hike that will cover 14 miles and have an elevation gain totaling 3,000 feet, you should allow yourself ten hours as a general rule.

Following the Blazes

Whether you spend a day hiking along its trails or half a year attempting to thru-hike its length, the Appalachian Trail's ever-present white blaze will follow you wherever you go. But what exactly are these blazes? Blazes verify that the hiker is indeed on the right track, and they mark the path the Trail takes through the woods.

At one time, blazes were made by gouging through a length of bark to the wood itself to mark the tree as a point-of-reference for the trail. Fortunately, blazes have become eco-friendly. Today, the Appalachian Trail is marked with white, rectangular paint blazes, though visitors will encounter other blazes along the A.T. (see page 176). In some areas, blazes are almost always within sight; in areas managed as wilderness you may encounter only four or five per mile. If you have hiked a quarter-mile without seeing a blaze, retrace your steps until you locate a blaze; then make sure you haven't missed a turn. Often a glance backwards will reveal additional blazes to help confirm your location.

To better protect the footpath, and to improve the quality of the backcountry experience, parts of the A.T. are occasionally relocated to cross recently acquired lands. Always follow the marked Trail. If it differs from your guidebook's Trail description, it is probably because the Trail was recently relocated in the area. Unless the old Trail has become a sanctioned blue-blazed alternate, following it may mean trespassing and generating ill will toward the Trail community.

Maps and guidebooks often contain information on pending relocations. For up-to-date information on current conditions, contact a local trail club or check the Appalachian Trail Conservancy's Web site for updates.

Taking Breaks

When we first started hiking, we took what we called a pack-off break every two miles and pack-on breaks after almost every hill. A pack-on or bend-over break is accomplished by leaning over and bracing your hands on your knees so that you shift the weight for a brief respite. Try it; it really helps when you first start hiking. By the time we had hiked 500 miles, we could hike for hours without any breaks at all.

TYPES OF BLAZES AND MARKERS

RECTANGULAR WHITE BLAZES (two inches wide by six inches tall): You will find these painted on trees, posts, or rocks. White-paint blazes provide continuous Trail marking from Maine to Georgia. They are the primary method of indicating the Trail route. In some areas you also may see diamond-shaped A.T. metal markers, which were a past form of marking the trail.

TWO RECTANGULAR WHITE BLAZES (one above the other, or with one slightly offset below the other): Found at obscure turns, route changes, or other situations requiring hiker alertness. You also may see the two blazes offset, indicating the direction of the turn.

RECTANGULAR BLUE BLAZES: Blue blazes mark the way to water, viewpoints, shelters, privies, and side trails from the A.T.

RECTANGULAR BLAZES IN OTHER COLORS: At some intersecting trails, you will find a different colored blaze indicating that another trail intersects the Appalachian Trail. While the trail may not be a part of the A.T., it might occasionally share the footpath.

OTHER BLAZES (irregular shapes, usually red or white): Found in National Forests and state game lands, these are boundary markers that hikers sometimes confuse with rectangular Trail blazes.

ROCK CAIRNS: These are often found above timberline, in fields and on balds, where no trees are available; a series of rock cairns (piles of rocks) are used to mark the Trail. Most are also marked with blazes. This makes the Trail visible even when snow- or fog-covered.

POSTS (with blazes): These can be found on balds, in farm pastures, and other treeless areas; also in national historical parks.

SIGNS: Signs are often found near shelters, road crossings, trail intersections, and water sources. Though A.T. managers keep signs to a minimum, you will see a few noting approximate hiking distances, identifying notable features, and providing safety information.

Taking breaks slows down your overall pace. One way to avoid frequent stops and keep up your pace is to use the rest step when ascending mountains. Perform the rest step by pausing for a moment with all your weight centered on your downhill leg, which should be kept straight. Then step forward and pause again with your weight on the opposite leg, which is now the downhill leg. Vary the length of the pause as needed. This step will not only get you up a steep slope sooner but will get you up a mountain with less effort.

The idea is to use this step on extremely tough sections of a hike by pausing slightly with each step—continual movement instead of vigorous hiking separated by a number of breaks.

But above all, listen to your body. If you start to get overheated, dizzy, or nauseous, then stop and rest. These could be signs of emerging problems (see heat-related illnesses, page 142) or a simple fact of overexertion. So, take a break. Better to reduce your pace than suffer an injury.

MINIMIZE YOUR IMPACT

In recent years "minimum-impact camping" has become the catchphrase for responsible outdoor etiquette. Groups, such as the Boy Scouts, who once espoused techniques like trenching around your tent to prevent water from running under it, have changed with the times and adopted low-impact techniques.

Minimum-impact camping is easily summarized by the National Park Service's advice as "Take nothing but pictures, leave nothing but footprints."

The following are measures you can, and should, take to eliminate any trace of your presence along the trail:

- Pack out all trash, including the tiniest bits of paper, plastic, gum, etc., both yours and that left by others.
- Limit your group size to six or less.
- Stay on the designated trail and walk single file; don't cut switchbacks.
- Camp in designated sites or well away from the trail; use sites that won't be harmed by your stay.
- Don't use soap in or near streams; keep pollutants away from water sources by camping at least 200 feet from lakes and streams.
- When washing yourself or your pots and dishes, carry water at least 200 feet

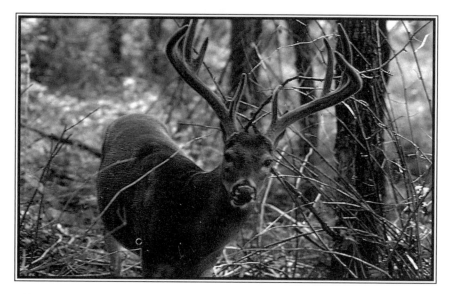

Buck along the A.T.

away from a water source. Sparingly use only biodegradable soap. and scatter dishwater.

- Always contain feces in a "cathole." Catholes must be six-to-eight-inches deep and at least 200 feet from water, camp, and trails. Cover and disguise hole when finished and pack out your toilet paper.
- Use a backpacking stove for cooking, a candle lantern or flashlight as a light source.
- Build fires only in designated fire pits, and use only downed wood; burn all wood or coal to ash; put out fires completely and scatter cool ashes.
- Be familiar with any regulations or special needs for the area where you intend to hike.
- Make sure you are familiar with any risks or dangers in the area where you are hiking.
- Do not damage historical structures or remove artifacts.
- Leave natural objects such as rocks and leaves where you found them.
- Do not build structures or dig trenches.
- Always observe wildlife from a distance; leave animals alone, particularly young animals and animals that are nesting or feeding.
- Never feed wild animals.
- Store food and other gear, including trash, well off the ground and out of animals' reach.
- Keep pets under control.
- Take breaks away from the Trail on durable surfaces.
- Keep noise level down.

This is a way of living that is becoming increasingly important to adopt. More than 4 million people hike some portion of the Appalachian Trail annually. If these techniques are not used by everyone (and currently they're not), the trail will lose its natural beauty. Nature is resilient but its ability to rebound from excessive use and mistreatment takes time. The damage from a single overnight stay by an inconsiderate group of hikers will linger long after the group has left.

When you leave a campsite, take a long, hard look at it. It should look better than when you found it. And if you camp off the Trail, the site you leave behind should look untouched. It can be done. We've even gone so far as to rescatter leaves and fluff up grass so that you could not tell that our tent had been pitched there. It only takes a few minutes and your efforts are more than compensated for with peace of mind.

PERMITS AND RESERVATIONS: WHERE ARE THEY NEEDED AND HOW TO GET THEM

Most places you hike along the A.T. require no special permission. You just get up and go. However, there are a few places where you need permission before hiking overnight. Permits are needed only within the National Park System, and in the case of the Appalachian Trail, in the Smokies and the Shenandoah. The heavy use of the A.T. in these areas has created a need to limit the number of hikers staying overnight in the parks. The permits are free and are used only to control the number of campers. Shelters in heavy-use areas—White Mountain National Forest (New Hampshire), Green Mountain National Forest (Vermont), and Baxter State Park (Maine)—often require a registration and/or fees.

GREAT SMOKY MOUNTAINS NATIONAL PARK (GSMNP)

A backcountry permit is required for all people spending the night in the park's backcountry, including the A.T. or its side trails. Backcountry permits may be obtained by mail or in person at all park campgrounds, ranger stations, and visitor centers.

Additionally, unless you are an A.T. thru-hiker, you must also reserve in advance a space in a specific shelter through the Park's Backcountry Reservations

Office; call (865) 436-1231, 8 a.m. to 4:30 p.m. or log on to **www.gsmnp.com.** Have your itinerary planned before you call. If, however, you are headed to the park to enjoy some day hikes, you may want to stay overnight in one of the park's many campsites. You may reserve these sites online at **http://reservations .nps.gov** or by phone at (800) 365-2267 (using the park code GRE).

In the Great Smokies, the term "thru-hiker" is defined as follows: A person who is hiking the entire length of the Appalachian Trail in a single trip; or a person who begins a hiking trip on the A.T. at least 50 miles outside the park, hikes the A.T. through the Smokies, and finishes the trip at least 50 miles outside the opposite boundary of the park. Thru-hikers are required to obtain a backcountry permit that allows seven consecutive nights and eight days to traverse the Trail, but are exempt from the reservation system. Because of the large number of northbound thru-hikers who enter the park between April 1 and June 15, three bunk spaces at each A.T. shelter are reserved for them during this time.

No more than one night may be spent at any one shelter. If a shelter you select for a night's stay has bunk space available, you must use it. However, if the shelter is full, a thru-hiker may set up camp within 50 feet of the shelter's front. No other tent camping is permitted on the A.T. in the Smokies.

During the spring thru-hiking season, it is quite likely that shelters will be overcrowded with thru-hikers, with numbers far exceeding the three spaces allotted at each shelter. If you encounter this situation, please be considerate of the other backpackers who may have reservations for the shelter, recognize their legitimate claim to their bunk space, and set up camp outside.

Northbound thru-hikers can obtain backcountry permits at the self-registration station at the Fontana Dam A.T. Shelter. Northbound thru-hikers cannot obtain permits by mail for travel between April 1 and June 15.

Southbound thru-hikers can obtain backcountry permits at the self-registration station near Big Creek Ranger Station or from the U.S. Forest Service office in Hot Springs, North Carolina, 33 miles north of Davenport Gap. Southbound hikers may also obtain permits by mail, regardless of when you plan to hike through the park. Getting caught by a ranger without a permit results in a fine (currently $125).

Reservations can be made in advance by calling (865) 436-1231 for permits; for trip planning information, call (865) 436-1297. If you have questions or require additional information, contact:

GREAT SMOKY MOUNTAINS NATIONAL PARK
107 Park Headquarters Road
Gatlinburg, TN 37738
(865) 436-1200 (visitor information recorded message)

SHENANDOAH NATIONAL PARK (SNP)

A permit is required for backcountry visitors in the park. Permits are available at park headquarters, all entrance stations, all campgrounds, all visitor centers, and at self-registration stations at either ends of the park: on the southern end at the park entrance on Skyline Drive, and on the northern end at 0.1 mile south of the park boundary sign.

Northbound thru-hikers can obtain backcountry permits at the self-registration station at the park entrance on Skyline Drive, accessible from the A.T. via a blue-blazed side trail 0.8 miles north of Rockfish Gap. Southbound thru-hikers can obtain backcountry permits at the self-registration station at Chester Gap, 0.1 mile south of the sign marking the park's northern boundary.

There is no charge for hikers entering the park via the Appalachian Trail. However, there is a $5 fee charged at some other trailheads, and a $10 per vehicle fee for entering via Skyline Drive. Permits are available only between the hours of sunrise and one hour before sunset. Permits may also be obtained by writing to the park superintendent (see below).

Huts (overnight shelters) are available on a first-come, first-serve basis. Long-distance hikers may tent near huts at designated sites if the huts are full. Campsites have been created and established by prior visitor use and are not posted or signed. You must camp at least 20 yards from a park trail or an unpaved fire road.

If you cannot locate a pre-existing campsite, you may camp on a previously undisturbed area. Please use "pristine site camping" practices to minimize the impact of your campsite. Limit your stay to one night and camp well out of sight of trails, roads, and camping groups. Otherwise, "pre-existing campsite" regulations apply.

Some campsites are park-constructed and posted to concentrate backcountry camping at specific high-use sites. Presently, designated campsites are provided only at Appalachian Trail huts to accommodate overflow camping.

Camping is allowed in park-constructed, designated campsites located at Appalachian Trail huts. Camping is also permitted in specific backcountry facilities. The Potomac Appalachian Trail Club (PATC) maintains a system of backcountry huts and cabins in Shenandoah National Park. Huts are three-sided structures located along the Appalachian Trail and operated by PATC for use by long-term hikers. Backcountry camping permits are required for camping in huts, and all park backcountry camping regulations apply. Permits are not required for cabins, which can be reserved in advance from PATC.

If you have questions or require additional information, contact:

Shenandoah National Park
3655 Highway 211 East
Luray, VA 22835
(540) 999-3500 (general information)

In Shenandoah National Park, No Camping May Occur:

- within ten yards of a stream or other natural water source;

- within 50 yards of standing building ruins, including stone foundations, chimneys, and log walls. The parkland has a rich cultural history; camping in the area of former homesites impacts the preservation of those resources;

- within 50 yards of another camping party or "no camping" post or sign or within a quarter mile of a paved road, park boundary, or park facility such as a campground, picnic area, visitor center, lodge, wayside, or restaurant;

- within 100 yards of a hut, cabin, or day-use shelter except when otherwise designated.

Green Mountain National Forest
(Vermont)

The Green Mountain Club (GMC) caretaker program is in effect throughout the hiking season, from early May through early November. A.T. hikers may find GMC caretakers at several sensitive, high-use overnight sites along the Trail. Through informal conversation and example, the caretakers educate hikers about "Leave No Trace"™ practices and perform Trail and shelter maintenance. A modest overnight fee is charged within a half mile of caretaker sites: $6 for non-members (reduced for GMC members), except at shelters on national forest land, where the discount is not allowed (fees subject to change). The shelter fees defray the cost of the GMC field programs and are used for Trail and shelter maintenance along the entire A.T. in Vermont, not just the fee sites.

As part of an effort to protect Vermont's alpine areas and fragile summits, the GMC also fields summit caretakers—on Stratton Mountain, Killington Peak, and Pico Peak. These caretakers talk with hikers about the fragile summit ecosystems, enforce camping and fire regulations, and provide first aid and assistance. At GMC pond sites—Stratton Pond, Griffith Lake, and Little Rock Pond along the A.T. in Vermont—a fee is charged for anyone camping within one-half mile of the body of water and campsite.

All shelters and campsites are available on a first-come basis. While dispersed camping is an option on national forest land in some areas of this section, hikers are encouraged to use backcountry facilities in order to lessen their impact on the Trail's environment.

Caretakers can be found, in season, at the following campsites:

Griffith Lake Tenting Area	Lula Tye Shelter
Little Rock Pond Campsite	North Shore Tenting Area
Little Rock Pond Shelter	Peru Peak Shelter
Lost Pond Shelter	Stratton Pond Shelter and Tentsites

A Green Mountain Club ridgerunner may be present at shelter sites along the Coolidge Range although a fee is not charged. Ridgerunners are present in some areas to protect the environment. They are there to make sure you are camping legally. For example, if you show up with a group of 20, they will make sure that you follow "Leave No Trace"™ rules. Sites with ridgerunners are:

Churchhill Scott Shelter	Minerva Hinchey Shelter
Clarendon Shelter	Pico Camp (still available to hikers although no longer on the A.T. due to a relocation)
Cooper Lodge	
Governor Clement Shelter	

Fees and regulations are subject to change. If you have questions or require additional information, contact:

GREEN MOUNTAIN CLUB
4711 Waterbury-Stowe Road
Waterbury Center, VT 05677
(802) 244-7037
www.greenmountainclub.org

GREEN MOUNTAIN NATIONAL FOREST
231 North Main Street
Rutland, VT 05701
(802) 747-6700
www.fs.fed.us/r9/gmfl

WHITE MOUNTAIN NATIONAL FOREST

(NEW HAMPSHIRE)

In recent years, use of backcountry trails and facilities in the White Mountains has increased dramatically. Soil erosion, loss of vegetation, water pollution, and disposal of human waste have become major problems, necessitating tougher regulations to lessen the impact from camping and hiking.

To prevent harming the forest's fragile ecosystems and to allow damaged areas to rehabilitate, the United States Forest Service has designated parts of the White Mountains as forest protection areas (FPAs). Camping and fires are restricted in FPAs; no camping is allowed above the treeline (where trees are at least eight feet tall); no camping is allowed within 200 feet of the Trail; and no camping is allowed within a quarter mile of any hut, shelter, or tentsite, except at the facility itself.

The A.T. passes through three state parks within the White Mountain National Forest: Franconia Notch State Park, Crawford Notch State Park, and the summit of Mount Washington. In these state parks, camping is permitted only in designated campgrounds, huts, or shelters. Camping is not permitted on Mount Washington's summit.

AMC TENTSITES, SHELTER, AND CAMPSITES

In the Whites, AMC maintains tentsites, shelters, campsites in addition to huts (see below), which are available on a first-come basis. Thru-hikers who wish to stay at any of AMC's facilities as paying guests will be offered the reduced club-member rate. Tentsites have designated tenting areas and platforms or pads and shelters are three- or four-sided structures. Campsites have tenting areas and a shelter.

Caretakers are in residence at the following tentsites, shelters, and campsites, and an $8 overnight fee is charged. All are located in New Hampshire:

Ethan Pond Campsite	Liberty Spring Tentsite
Garfield Ridge Campsite	Nauman Tentsite
Guyot Campsite	Speck Pond Campsite
Imp Campsite	13 Falls Tentsite
Kinsman Pond Campsite	

The remaining tentsites, shelters, and campsites are available to backcountry travelers at no charge.

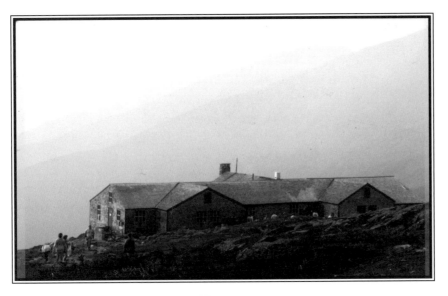

Lakes of the Clouds hut in New Hampshire

AMC HUTS

These large, enclosed structures sleep from 36 to 90 people and provide various amenities during the full-service season (from the first Friday in June to September or October, depending on the hut) and are closed the rest of the year. (Exceptions include Carter Notch and Crawford, which are self-service year-round, and Zealand, which is self-service October through May. These huts have only a caretaker, with lower rates for self-service stays.) A crew staffs the facilities during the full-service season. The overnight rate is $75 (for a non-AMC member adult), and includes bunk space, pillow, blanket, rest-room privileges (no showers), and potable water. Thru-hikers staying as paying guests will be offered the club's 10-percent member discount whether they are members or not. If you plan to stay three consecutive nights, there is a package rate of $53 per night. A one-night stay for thru-hikers at Lonesome Lake Hut is also $50 per night. Caretaker rates at any of the facilities is $20. Each hut has trained wilderness EMTs and First Responders, and the facilities crew gives natural- and cultural-history evening programs. The huts also contain excellent libraries and displays of cultural and natural history.

If you plan to pay for a stay in one of the huts, make reservations, (603) 466-2727, especially on the weekends, when bunk spaces fill quickly. The huts cater mainly to families and weekend hikers. AMC recently had wells drilled at all the huts, so you can look forward to water that meets state health standards.

Thru-hikers can sometimes arrange with the crew to work off their stays. Most huts can accommodate one or two working thru-hikers each night, but availability of work is never guaranteed. This work exchange is on a first-come basis. Work varies, but you can expect to put in two to four hours in the morning. Lakes of the Clouds Hut takes up to four thru-hikers.

During the self-service season, guests must bring their own sleeping bags, and hikers have access to the kitchen and cookware to prepare meals. The self-service rates start at $23 for members, $25 for nonmembers.

For current information on this area, contact:

WHITE MOUNTAIN NATIONAL FOREST
Forest Supervisor
P.O. Box 638
Laconia, NH 03246
(603) 528-8721
www.fs.fed.us/r9/white

APPALACHIAN MOUNTAIN CLUB
Pinkham Notch Visitors Center
Route 16
P.O. Box 298
Gorham, NH 03581
(603) 466-2721 (general information)
(603) 466-2727 (hut reservations, 9 a.m. –5 p.m. , Monday–Saturday)
www.outdoors.org

BAXTER STATE PARK (MAINE)

Baxter State Park (where Katahdin is located) was designed to value resource preservation over recreation. Most of its rules and policies stem from either that philosophy or the weather. Unlike the surrounding landscape below, Katahdin is exposed to extreme weather, including high winds and is capable of receiving snow every month of the year. There are no shelters located above treeline and all trails to the summit are completely exposed. On humid, late-summer days, it is wise to start down from the mountain by 1 p.m. to avoid electrical storms.

The park is open for general use from May 15 to October 15. From October 15 to December 1, and from April 1 to May 15, the park is open for day use. From December 1 to April 1, camping, climbing, and mountain hiking are allowed only by special-use permit, for which application must be made to Park Headquarters in Millinocket at least two weeks in advance.

Fees are charged for the use of all shelters and tent space. Camping is permitted only in authorized campgrounds. All persons entering or leaving the park by way of the A.T. no longer register at the Daicey Pond Campground. There is now a kiosk a mile north of Abol Bridge.

Long-distance hikers planning to stay in Baxter State Park should be aware of the following:

UNTIL OCTOBER 15: The park's site for distance hikers is "The Birches" near Katahdin Stream Campground. Thru-hikers without reservations may stay at this site (limited to one-night stay), which has a maximum capacity of 12 (two four-person lean-tos and one tent platform; park-wide fee applies.) If there is no room at the Birches, you may stay at Katahdin Stream Campground, which has no thru-hiker designated sites, but you may check with any ranger for availability of a regular public site (at regular fee). Availability is least likely in August and on fall weekends, most likely mid-week after Labor Day.

AFTER OCTOBER 15: There is no overnight camping anywhere within the park so you will need to camp at the private Abol Bridge Campground or the Abol Pines Campsite just downriver of Abol Bridge. Both sites charge fees. There are no other options for authorized overnight camping near the Trail after October 15. Your hike to the summit is thus 15 miles (one way) from this area outside the park. Most late hikers stay in a motel in Millinocket instead, and hire a taxi to shuttle them in and out of the park on the day of their hike.

No special permission is required for day use below tree line. However, in the interest of public safety, the park strongly discourages people from traveling alone in the winter, and a party size of at least two is strongly recommended—three or four is better! Day users are requested to check in and out at park gates, volunteer registration points, Park Headquarters, or by phone if more convenient. This is for the safety of users in the event of an accident or emergency and helps them keep statistics on park use.

A note to southbounders: Katahdin is a tough climb. The footpath below tree line is more rocks and roots than soil. Above tree line, you pull yourself over rocks in a few places and walk across slanted, roof-sized boulders in others. The climb is hard enough without a pack. Northbounders and southbounders alike should leave their packs at the ranger station at Katahdin Stream Campground. Bring a daypack or fanny pack with water, snacks, sunscreen, and warm clothing for the summit.

For more information:

BAXTER STATE PARK
64 Balsam Drive
Millinocket, ME 04462
(207) 723-5140
www.baxterstateparkauthority.com

GUIDEBOOKS

T he Appalachian Trail Conservancy offers a number of books that can help you with planning and carrying out a hike.

THE APPALACHIAN TRAIL
GUIDEBOOK SERIES

This series of 11 books offers detailed trail descriptions for both north-to-south and south-to-north hikes. The books provide information on mileage between major points, shelters and facilities on the trail, road crossings and trailhead parking, water, side trails, and relevant history of the area the trail is passing through.

All of the guidebooks come with 3 to 12 maps. The topographic maps also include elevation profiles, which should not be taken literally: flat sections on the elevation profile are almost never truly level when you are actually hiking the trail. And some steep sections, especially those on the Maine maps, are not quite as bad as they appear on the profile.

The Appalachian Trail is well blazed, and a detailed, step-by-step description is not necessary to keep from getting lost. The trail descriptions do, however, keep you informed of your progress and how far it is to the next shelter, water, etc.

Guidebooks cannot be taken as Gospel. The trail route gets altered, storms knock down trees, springs dry up and disappear, and the trail descriptions are the opinions of the writer. The guides are updated every couple of years or so. They can be purchased with the maps or you can buy the maps separately.

You can also purchase the trail guides on CD-ROM. Ten of the eleven Appalachian Trail guide sets, including books and maps (trail guides for half of Pennsylvania are produced by The Keystone Trails Association) are available on four CD-ROMs with a free strip map of the whole Trail, plus Maptech's Terrain Navigator planning software.

APPALACHIAN TRAIL DATA BOOK

The *Appalachian Trail Data Book* is updated annually to keep hikers current with the relocations of the Trail. It contains mileages between points on the Trail. At road crossings, the *Data Book* lists distances to post offices, lodgings, groceries, and restaurants.

This book informs you of the location of shelters and notes if the shelter doesn't have water available. It also lets you know the distance between sources of water in water-scarce areas.

The ATC intended the *Data Book* to be used only for broad-scale planning of hikes; but it is also a practical guide that can be taken along with you (or a photocopy of the pages you need), particularly if you opt not to carry the Trail guidebooks.

The *Appalachian Trail Mate*, a CD-ROM version of the *A.T. Data Book*, is also available with trip-planning software included, developed under license from the ATC.

THE APPALACHIAN TRAIL THRU-HIKER'S COMPANION

This small book published annually by the Appalachian Trail Conservancy offers a wealth of information to long-distance hikers on goods and services available along the Trail and much more. The guide is edited by the Appalachian Long-Distance Hikers Association. The book is compiled for the following spring from information supplied by thru-hikers and others at the end of every year. This spiral-bound book will help you decipher the information in the *Data Book* by telling you more about the places, such as grocery stores, than the letter code in the *Data Book* conveys.

Another, non-ATC, guide available for thru-hikers is Dan Bruce's *The Thru-hiker's Handbook*, which is also updated annually. It is available from Bruce at **www.trailplace.com**.

FINDING SOLITUDE

Many hikers retreat to the Appalachian Trail seeking a wilderness experience, only to find themselves on a crowded section of trail sharing their "wilderness experience" with more hikers than they bargained for. Here are a few tips for finding a little solitude on America's most popular long-distance trail.

Start your hike early in the morning. We once took this advice to the extreme and enjoyed the best hike of our lives for the effort. We started climbing Katahdin at 2:30 a.m. and were up at Baxter Peak by 5:30 a.m. for the sunrise. The view was spectacular, and the three of us hiking together didn't share the summit with another hiker. That was on Labor Day weekend, when later in the day hikers marched in a long single file from Baxter Peak to Pamola Peak. By making an extra effort to get up early (and hike the tricky section of Trail in the dark), we had the peak to ourselves on perhaps the busiest day of the year.

Another way to find your own piece of the A.T. is to go during the off-season. Roan Highlands on the Tennessee–North Carolina state line is very crowded during the peak bloom time for the rhododendron garden. Visitors flock to see the awesome spectacle of thousands of catawba rhododendrons in bloom. But we have camped alone on the summit during the winter. We couldn't see the rhododendron blooms that attract the big crowds, but the mountain covered in fresh snow was a magnificent sight, and we didn't have to share it with hoards of hikers.

The third way to find solitude on the country's most popular long-distance trail is to find your own special places. There are a number of very popular areas on the A.T. from Blood Mountain in Georgia and Shenandoah National Park in Virginia to Katahdin in Maine, as well as many others. Most of the use of the trail is concentrated in these easy-to-access spots, while many other areas go unappreciated. Join a trail club in your area and learn from other members and group hikes where some of the less visited areas are.

If you are planning a thru-hike but still want the option of solitude, try leaving Springer Mountain before March 1 or after mid-April. Southbound hikes, flip-flops and leapfrogs are other options that will be discussed in the chapter on long-distance hiking.

Hiking downhill is as tough on your body as an uphill climb. Whereas an ascent places cardiovascular stress on your body, a descent takes its toll on your feet and knees. To lessen the impact try pausing with your weight on one foot between each step; this will relieve some of the strain. Also, spring forward with each step, flexing your legs as you put weight on them. This is the fastest and safest way to get downhill.

Chapter Twelve

Winter Backpacking

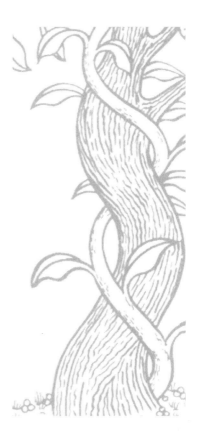

Snows in the north Georgia mountains are so rare that you have to keep an eye on the Weather Channel if you want to hike in more than an inch. So, when Frank and I heard that the north Georgia mountains were going to receive several inches of snow, we planned an impromptu day hike. We piled into our Jeep with our friends, Joe and Monica Cook, and our daughter, Griffin, and headed for the hills.

In four-wheel drive, we labored up the forest service road to the base of Springer Mountain, the southern terminus of the Appalachian Trail. Seeing your favorite spots encrusted and powdered with snow is like walking in an entirely different world. Thrilled with the first hike, we headed down to Three Forks to see what kind of fairy kingdom the snow had made down there. It was an idyllic scene. Noontootla Creek burbled along as if it were an ordinary day, but the rhododendron on its banks were frosted with an icing of snow, and even the exposed stones in the creek boasted an inch or two of powder.

Experienced hikers have learned that pleasurable hiking need not only be found during the spring, summer, and fall. Winter camping is possible in many parts of the United States and provides much more solitude. It is a way to experience the Earth during its darkest season—to discover a new world both physically and mentally.

Even in the south, where contrary to popular opinion, it does get cold and even snows, you'll find the trails much less crowded. By the same token, you can find snowy places throughout the country where you can hike and camp in peace. And, of course, you don't have to hike in the snow. The cold, alone, can be enough to keep many hikers off the trail.

Before you throw on your pack and snow-seal your boots, keep in mind that winter backpacking requires a little more forethought as well as preparation. You must decide whether you intend to hike in boots (with or without crampons), on snowshoes, or on cross-country skis. If the snow is not deep or if it is hard-packed, boots will probably suffice. A pair of gaiters and well-sealed boots will make the trip more comfortable. The hard, plastic, cold-weather mountaineering boots which were designed for technical climbing are impractical for backpacking.

GETTING AROUND:
EQUIPMENT FOR YOUR FEET

CRAMPONS

While three-season hikers, including A.T. thru-hikers, will never need them, some winter backpacking on the A.T. requires the use of crampons. This is particularly true in the White Mountains. Simply put, crampons are a device you strap onto your boots that help give you good footing on ice and hard snow.

Crampons must be fitted properly—loose crampons can be more danger-ous than hiking crampon-less across slick ice or snow. For backpacking, flexible crampons are a must. Consult an outdoor retailer that features climbing equip-ment when choosing a pair. You will also need to have the proper boot. Not all boots will accept crampons.

Another option for winter hiking (including late-season thru-hikers) is to use the smaller and lighter instep crampons, which sell for less than $10 per pair.

When hiking with crampons, an ice axe is another useful piece of equip-ment. It will help you cut steps in ice or snow and can be used as a brake to stop yourself should you fall. The purchase of an ice ax should be discussed with your local outfitter.

THE ICE AXE

This tool is designed with a pointed end (the spike) and a head consisting of a spoon-shaped blade called the adze at one end and a long and narrow blade at the other end of the head called the pick. Some winter hikers get double use out of the ice axe by using it as a hiking stick, too.

Its main use, though, is to assist in slowing a fall or slide down an icy slope. To ensure your safety, you'll need to learn the self-arrest technique.

ICE-AXE SELF-ARREST

When learning the self-arrest technique without an actual instructor, keep in mind that the most dangerous thing is dropping down onto your "slope" and gouging yourself in the face with the axe. So, before you drop, concentrate fiercely on holding the adze away from your face. You don't want to be sitting in the emergency room saying, "Yeah, I was practicing how not to hurt myself. . ."

Also keep in mind that when self arresting only three things will come in contact with the ground—the pick of the axe, your left foot, and your right foot. Your body should be off the ground and your legs should be spread, somewhat, to form a triangle and provide you with some lateral stability.

Are you ready to try it? In your backyard (or wherever you are practicing):

- Lie down on the ground and fix your body in the self-arrest position. That is, spread your legs and brace your body off the ground using your toes and the adze (which is well away from your face, remember) for support.
- Memorize this position.
- Next, find an actual slope (with snow, if it's available) that you can practice on without hurting yourself. Don't get all gung ho and practice on a steep slope where you might end up in the hospital.

- Once again, when you fall, don't forget to keep a tight grip on the axe and to keep that adze AWAY from your face.
- Use your stronger arm to hold the ice axe. Should you actually fall on an icy snow slope, you are not going to have time to think about what you need to do. The self-arrest will have to be a reflex action.
- When you are practicing falling, make sure you practice falling when you are climbing up the slope as well as practicing falling when you are descending.
- Never switch hands—always hold the ice axe with the same hand.
- If you slip and land on your back or bottom, roll over onto your stomach in the direction AWAY from the spike of your axe. This way, the spike won't catch in the snow as you roll over. If you are right-handed, for example, you would roll to the left.

SNOWSHOES

Much of the A.T. can be walked in the winter in hiking boots. However, the snow gets deep in the mountains of New England (even in the mid-Atlantic and Southern states at times), and snowshoes are a fun way to stay on top of the snow. Snowshoes with crampons on the bottoms are advantageous when it comes to climbing steep slopes, even on crusty or icy snow. Climbing can be extremely tiring, though, especially at high altitudes. Breaking trail is also difficult in snowshoes—difficult and exhausting—particularly if the snow is wet and heavy or more than a foot deep. Each step requires that you raise your foot high enough to clear the snow surface. If you're going to be breaking trail, use larger snowshoes with as much flotation as possible.

Trade off leaders every half hour or so to keep the trailbreaker from becoming too exhausted or overheated. When taking the lead, always take into consideration the pace of the slowest member of the group and make your steps short enough so everyone in the group can follow in them. Those following should stay in the leader's footsteps whenever possible. Not only is it easier going but it leaves a more well-defined trail for your return trip or for others who follow you. Remember, though, that even with snowshoes, four hours a day is about all most hikers can manage to backpack in the snow.

It can be difficult to sort out the pair of snowshoes you need from the many options available on the market. But with some general guidelines to follow, you can select the best snowshoes to match your needs and the terrain and snow conditions in which you will be hiking.

The frame will be made of aluminum tubing, wood, or plastic. Frames vary according to the shape. The Yukon is a long snowshoe with the traditional teardrop shape that tapers out into a tail; the tail helps you track or stay on a

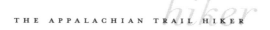

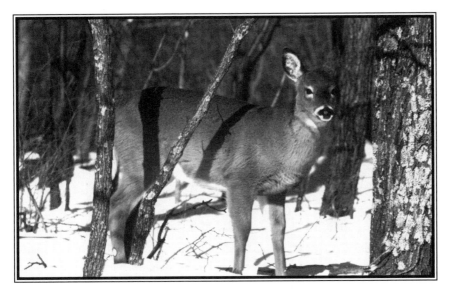

Snow on the A.T., Shenandoah National Park, Virginia

straight line in deep powder. The Western style is an elongated oval that is quite popular, and the Green Mountain bearpaw design is a hybrid that works in a variety of conditions. Wider snowshoes are ideal for soft, deep snow, while a narrow snowshoe is preferable for sidehill walking. An upturned toe makes downhill walking easier.

Snowshoe decks have evolved from the traditional cowhide webbing deck. Lightweight materials, including polyurethane-coated nylon, vinyl, and Hypalon give superior flotation to smaller-sized snowshoes. For backcountry use, you will also be shopping for snowshoes that come with built-in toe crampons. The crampons will give the shoes the grip they need when climbing or when traversing icy snow.

An important consideration with snowshoes is the binding that attaches the snowshoe to your boots. Bindings range from simple leather straps to a complicated harness made of high-performance Hypalon. What matters most is how well the bindings fit your boots and how comfortable they are to wear. The only way to find out is to try them on. The best way to check out binding fit is to rent a pair to try before you buy. As you try on the bindings, notice if they pinch or bind. Do they rub your foot as you walk? These problems only get worse over time. Look for the best possible fit to eliminate problems in the backcountry.

The overall size of the snowshoes depends on your size and the snow conditions in which you anticipate hiking. Snowshoe sizes fall into three main categories: 8 x 25 inches, 9 x 30 inches, and 10 x 36 inches. These sizes are approximate with manufacturers creating their own unique designs. Larger snowshoes are needed for deep powder, and smaller shoes are acceptable for compacted or wet snow. Smaller snowshoes are for smaller hikers, with 8 x 25-inch designs working well for hikers under 175 pounds. Keep in mind, though, that the weights refer to the combined weight of the hiker and full pack. The 10 x 30-inch designs work for combined weights over 225 pounds. The 9 x 30-inch snowshoes are generally for hikers who fall between 175 and 225 pounds. Those hiking frequently on deep powder may want to opt for one-size-larger shoe.

Sorel, or other insulated boots, are worn with snowshoes to keep your feet dry and warm. Be sure to wear your hiking or snowshoeing boots when trying on snowshoes. That way you will ensure a proper fit with the snowshoe bindings. A pair of ski poles can be of assistance in snowshoeing as well as skiing (many back-packers use ski poles as hiking sticks). A good book on the subject is *Snowshoeing: From Novice to Master* by Gene Prater (published by The Mountaineers).

OTHER WINTER EQUIPMENT

TENT

If you're heading out into the snow, you'll need a four-season tent, preferably one that offers a cookhole in its floor. In the deep South, a three-season tent will probably suffice at all but the highest altitudes, since the temperature rarely drops below 20 °F. Whatever tent you use, it should have a waterproof floor.

A freestanding tent is the best choice for snow camping. Non-freestanding tents need special pegs to keep the tent anchored in the snow and they don't always work. A freestanding tent doesn't need to be anchored except in strong winds. Special tent anchors for snow camping can be purchased from most out-doors stores. Once your tent is anchored, try pouring some water on the pegs. Once it freezes, the pegs really won't move.

Some four-season tents offer cookholes: a zippered or gathered hole in the bottom of the tent floor that can be flapped or pulled back so that you may cook directly on the ground. A cookhole is preferable to cooking on the floor of your tent, which can catch fire easily should the stove tip. Fumes and the danger of starting a fire are potential problems. You should only cook in the tent itself if weather dictates. Cooking in the vestibule is generally a safer option.

When pitching your tent in the snow, make sure you level the area and pack down the snow. If this is not done, it is very likely you will wake up when the tent collapses on your head as the heat of your body will have collapsed the snow under you, changed the contours of the ground, and caused the properly pitched tent to sag. Leaving your pack on while you stamp the ground flat will give you some extra weight that will make the job go more quickly. If you make the base wider than necessary, you'll be able to walk around your tent without snowshoes or skis, especially useful should nature call in the middle of the night.

THE CALL OF NATURE AND SNOW

If you are camping in deep snow or on frozen earth, you can't bury your excrement in the snow, because as soon as the snow melts, there it will sit for all the world to see. You will have to carry out your excrement. Double-bag it in zipper-lock-style bags, pack it away from food items, and dispose of it properly at the end of your trip.

SLEEPING BAG

When camping during the winter, you will also need a sleeping bag with a high comfort rating—a zero-degree bag will do for most situations. If you don't want the expense of two sleeping bags, consider using a liner to make your three-season bag warmer. It should go without saying that you will need a mummy-style bag for winter camping. Mummy bags fit more closely to your body than square-cut bags, offering better insulating ability. Also, with less cold air coming into the open end of the bag, the mummy bags keep you warmer. If the temperature really drops, you can tighten the hood until nothing but your nose is showing. Some sleeping bags are available with extra insulation in the foot of the bag to combat cold feet.

Since the bottom of your tent may be on top of snow, you will want some good insulation between the bottom of your tent and yourself. While a three-quarters-length sleeping pad may do for three-season camping, if your feet get cold easily you may want to consider a full-length pad for winter camping.

Cold-weather Clothing

Remember that layering your clothing is of utmost importance when backpacking during the winter. Beginning with a layer of long underwear, you may want to add a warm shirt and pants, or a pile or fleece shirt and pants set. You can top these off with a layer that includes a warm parka and waterproof, insulated pants if it is really cold or a rain/wind suit if the temperature is only reasonably cold. Don't forget that you can add greatly to your warmth by donning a hat or balaclava.

If you are sufficiently bundled, the exertion of hiking should keep you warm. If you start feeling hypothermic, stop immediately, change into dry clothes if yours are wet, crawl into your sleeping bag, and drink some hot liquid. Make sure the stove you bring will light (as well as boil water) in frigid weather.

Remember that when hiking on open snow, it is wise to wear sunglasses because the sun reflecting off the bright, white snow can burn your eyes. Snow-blindness can occur even on overcast days. If you don't have sunglasses, cut eye-slits in anything (a bandana, for example) that can tie around your head. Should someone become snowblind, cold compresses, a painkiller, and a lightproof bandage are needed. About 18 to 20 hours later, the blindness should fade.

WATER

You won't sweat as much in the winter, but your body is still using fluids and you will need to drink steadily to keep your body replenished. Here are a few important tips that relate to water when hiking in snow or cold weather:

Never drink icy water in the winter or even on cool days. The cold water can cause your body temperature to drop. To avoid this, warm snow or water in your mouth before swallowing.

Protect your water when temperatures drop below freezing by burying it deep in your pack. At night, stash it inside your tent or at the end of your sleeping bag. You can also turn your water bottles upside down so that ice won't block the spout.

When hiking in deep snow, you can keep your bottles full of water by topping off with snow after each drink.

Use water to melt snow. An inch of water in your cook pot will melt snow more quickly. Add the crustiest, iciest, or wettest snow to your pot—it will produce more water.

Keep in mind that melting snow will take more fuel and more time. With a cold wind blowing, it can take an hour and a stove full of fuel to melt and boil a quart of water.

It probably goes without saying to heed the words of Frank Zappa and avoid yellow snow, but also steer clear of pink or "watermelon" snow. This snow gets its name from its color, taste, and scent produced by microorganisms that can cause diarrhea.

All of the equipment needed for winter camping—warm clothes, four-season tents, sleeping bags, tent anchors, snowshoes, or skis—is available through outdoor retailers where you will also find information on how to use the equipment.

When hiking in snow, rotate the trail-breaking duty among the hikers. It is easy to let yourself get tired and possibly careless if you push too hard.

Chapter Thirteen

Backpacking with Children

When we decided to take a backpacking trip along the A.T. to Grayson Highlands in Virginia, we told our daughter that she would probably see a number of wild ponies. She was thrilled. All the way from Georgia to Virginia, she repeated over and over, "Mama see wild horse, Papa see wild horse, Griffin see wild horse."

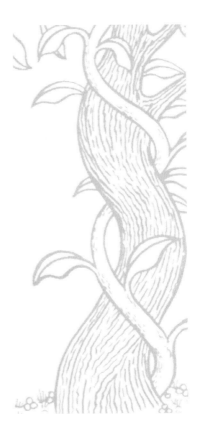

When we finally settled Griffin in her backpack, I began to experience some trepidation. What if we didn't see any wild ponies? Griffin was so excited that I felt like a horse myself, as she urged me on, heels pressing into my ribs.

I had nothing to fear. We had hiked less than 100 yards when we spied our first pony. From that point on, we nearly swam through ponies. When we set up camp, we soon had ponies surrounding our tent, nosing our backpacks, testing the strength of tent poles with their teeth. One pony, much to Griffin's delight, stuck her head in our tent.

Later, Griffin and I frolicked along with two young foals, racing along the grassy meadows of the Highlands. That night, as a sliver of a moon rose in the west, Griffin drifted off to sleep to the sound of thundering hooves, whickers, and neighs.

For parents, the question often arises: Should you take your children hiking and backpacking on the A.T.?

Why not? Most children love the outdoors. I have vivid memories of camping with my family in the mountains of California that have led me to continue my love affair with nature.

I discovered my daughter's love for the outdoors when she was three months old. While attending a conference in San Diego, I found that Griffin fell asleep more quickly when I carried her around outside than she did when I walked her in our room. Maybe it was all those long walks I took trying to induce labor when she was two weeks overdue, but she blossoms when the wind caresses her face and the sun shines on her head. She even loves the sprinkle of rain and overcast skies!

From carrying a child in a pack, one can advance to having the child carry a pack, increasing the pack size and weight carried as the child grows. Griffin can now backpack with the best of them.

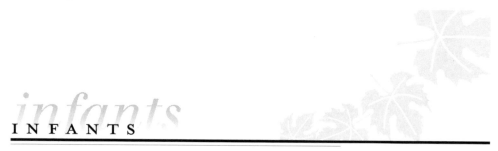

INFANTS

The younger the child is, the more difficult the packing (except for ages four to six months when they have not yet learned to crawl). Younger than four months, they don't yet fit in a pack, and after six months, they take off as soon as they touch the ground. If possible, set up your tent before you put your child down; you will have a handy playpen to hold the child until you've set up camp.

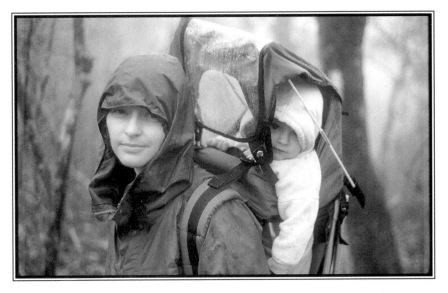

Victoria Logue with her daughter, Griffin

Until the child is toilet-trained, you must carry diapers—disposable or otherwise. You'll have to pack them in and out. Cindy Ross suggests cloth diapers which she and her husband, Todd, dry on the back of their packs so that they are lighter to carry. When the child has a bowel movement, you can simply bury her poop as you would your own, fold up the diaper, and carry it in a sealable plastic bag.

Because one person is carrying the child, the amount of extra stuff that person can carry is limited. This means the length of your trip is shortened, though there are ways to get around that.

One option is to plan a hike where you know you'll be able to stop at stores often enough to pick up the items you'll need—more food and diapers. Another option is to send extra items to post offices along the way if you have steady access to them. Finally, there is the option of a support crew that meets you at road crossings with the extra things you need.

As for food, once the child has started on solids, it will make your trip a bit more difficult until she can eat what you eat without mashing, smashing, etc. If you plan meals that your child can eat, too, then you can bring along a hand grinder. Also, some health food stores offer dehydrated baby foods. Jars of baby food are an option, but are heavy and will not keep very long once the jar is opened.

If your child is still breastfeeding but not yet on solids, you're in a perfect situation for backpacking because you don't have to carry formula and bottles. Although difficult, using formula is not impossible. Bottles can be heated on your cook stove the same way they would be heated on your stove at home—by warming them in water in your cook pot.

As for clothes, you know your child best. Your child may not need as many layers as another baby. It is best to remain aware of your child's needs and to respond to them. Children can be layered as easily as adults. There are plenty of manufacturers now, such as Backcountry, Gramicci, and Patagonia, who provide a range of layering options for children. Many catalogs even offer miniature rain suits.

Keep in mind that there are many things infants under six months of age cannot do—such as wear sunscreen or insect repellent. If you are hiking in the sun, they need a wide-brimmed hat or a screen on their backpack. If your infant will wear them, there are sunglasses available in infant sizes. While still an infant, Griffin successfully wore the Flap-happy Hat sold by Biobottoms of California. The baseball-style cap had a wide front brim and a protective flap of material that covered her delicate neck. Patagonia makes a similar hat for infants and children.

When it comes time to bed down for the night, where do you put your infant? When Griffin was younger, I shared my bag with her but she is now too big for that. I have yet to find an infant-sized sleeping bag although some companies make bags designed to keep an infant warm that work well as sleeping bags. You may also want to try designing your own with a child-size down comforter or several blankets.

Some children have no trouble falling asleep in a dark tent while others who wake to total darkness will freak-out. Keep a flashlight handy should you need to comfort your child with a little light. Others may find the confining walls of a tent disconcerting and fuss, but usually they get used to a tent after a night or two.

Keep in mind that a two-person tent is too small for the three of you, while a three-person tent will suit you for a long time.

I am only mentioning one child at this point; unless your second, third, etc. child can carry her own pack or hike entirely on her own, your backpacking will be limited to day hikes, though llama packing is an option in some areas.

TODDLERS

While you have basically the same concerns while backpacking with a toddler as you do with an infant, there is one major difference—toddlers can walk.

Unfortunately, hiking for a toddler means two entirely different methods of movement: 1) Running, which usually ends up with the child on his face, especially on unlevel trails; and 2) Walking a few steps and then stopping to explore, walking a few steps then stopping to explore, walking a few . . . .

Both of these styles can result in frustration for the parent but are absolutely necessary for the sanity of your child. As much as your child may love riding on your back in a backpack carrier, they still need to get out of it every once in awhile to stretch their legs.

This means that they'll be eager to escape from your pack and hit the ground running. Once toddlers are out of the pack, they demand at least one set of eyes on them constantly. The outdoors is great for growing minds, but also poses certain dangers, especially if the child is still teething; everything she picks up is likely to end up in her mouth. She needs you to keep her from eating poison ivy, snails, deer droppings, etc.

Most packs for child carrying will hold your toddler until he reaches 35 to 40 pounds. After that, you will begin backpacking with . . .

CHILDREN

This will be a difficult stage, no doubt about it. Your child—even packless—will walk a hundred yards (if you're lucky) and then start complaining, weeping, and wailing that he is tired. Remember that this is the same kid who can easily run the length of three football fields while playing with his friends.

When your child is at this stage, it is best to take frequent breaks until you reach your destination. You are thus limited to the number of miles you pack each day. No problem—just tone down your trips for awhile.

Your child can start with a fanny or daypack and carry his own toys and clothing. As your child gets older and stronger, you can move on to bigger packs and add food and a sleeping bag to the gear he is carrying.

GEAR

Outdoor gear manufacturers discovered children in the 1990s. The amount of kid gear on the market steadily increased during that decade and continues.

Mummy-designed sleeping bags rated for 15 °F can be purchased for children up to 48 inches. Manufacturers making kid bags include Feathered Friends, Eastern Mountain Sports, Peak 1, REI, and The North Face.

There are also packs designed especially for children as well as for parents who carry their children. Tough Traveler, Gerry, and Kelty all make superb packs to carry your infant or toddler. Designed to hold kids up to 35 or 40 pounds, all include a pocket to carry diapers and other essentials. An optional rain/sunscreen and extra pockets can be purchased with the Tough Traveler.

Children's packs are made by a number of manufacturers, including Tough Traveler, REI, Kelty, Jansport, and Osprey.

Manufacturers also offer children's hiking boots. Vasque, Hi-Tec, Tecnica, and others make hiking boots starting at about children's size ten. You can even find little boots for toddlers, but make sure they can actually walk in them before you purchase them for your child—they may be absolutely adorable but too rigid for a toddler's intrepid step.

MOTIVATING CHILDREN

How can you make backpacking fun for your children and avoid the "how much farther" syndrome? The following are a few suggestions:

- **REVEL IN NATURE.** Stop to point out interesting flowers, clouds, trees, mushrooms, etc. Enjoy water by throwing pebbles, floating sticks and leaves. Play in sand or mud or snow. Watch frogs hop, squirrels and chipmunks scuttle from tree to tree, insects crawling about, a deer standing stock still, a hawk drifting on air currents . . .

- **TEACH YOUR CHILDREN GEOLOGIC AND NATURAL HISTORY**—that Native Americans once hunted in these woods, that you are walking on what was once hot lava, about the intricacies of the glacier that molded this valley . . .

- **ANSWER YOUR CHILD'S QUESTIONS:** "Why is the sky blue?" "Are there still Indians in these woods?" "Will the volcano erupt on us?" . . .

- **GET OUT THE TOYS AND A TREAT.** Give your child a break with some fruit leather or a muffin and his favorite toy.

- **PROMISE A CELEBRATION WHEN THEY HAVE ATTAINED A CERTAIN GOAL.** Give them some juice and a piece of candy or cookie when they reach the top of the mountain or the next stream.

- **PLAY GAMES THAT KEEP YOU MOVING.** On slight declines play Runaway Train by running wildly to the bottom of the hill (only if your child is capable of doing this without falling on his face); continue the train theme by pretending your family is a train, making the appropriate noises while walking. Try some other vehicle—airplane, ship, racecar, truck.

- **TELL STORIES.** Tell stories of past but true events, make up stories, or even invite the children to tell a story. Asking questions can also prolong children's stamina.

- **SING SONGS.** Let the child choose or take turns choosing.

- **PLAY ANIMALS.** Pick an animal and tell about it, makes its noises, etc.

- **GIVE THEM GORP.** A handful of gorp for every 5, 10, 15, 20 steps (or whatever they're capable of) will keep them going for awhile.

At some point or another your child will pull the "I can't take another step with-out collapsing" trick. When the parent falls for this ploy and the child is carried to your destination, the little one usually experiences a miracle upon arrival. The child's eyes spring open and she's off and running while the poor, exhausted parents later have to beg her to crawl into her sleeping bag.

On the other hand, children do not recognize fatigue and will drop from exhaustion before they show any true signs of tiring. Children are tough but not superhuman. Don't push them too hard. Chances are, if you're tired, so are they.

If you want to get your children motivated before they hike, you might want to get a copy of the *Appalachian Trail Fun Book*. The coloring and activity book introduces four- to nine-year-olds to the A.T. It's published by the Appalachian Trail Conservancy, and available through them, as well as in book-stores and backpacking shops.

LIMITATIONS

Unless one partner is capable of carrying most of the gear (or in the case of a walking child, the parents can split most of the gear) you will have to put off any major backpacking trips until your child is old enough to take care of himself.

A single parent will have to limit backpacking trips to day hikes unless they intend to camp extra light (which is not really wise if you're hiking with children) by not carrying a tent, cookstove, etc.

You should be aware of your own limitations. If you can't regularly carry a 60-pound pack, don't think that you can do it if you have a child. If you normally carry a 40-pound pack and your child weighs 20 pounds, carry no more than 20 pounds of gear, for a total weight of 40 pounds of child and equipment. Remember, you have a life on your back now. Don't endanger it.

Introducing your child to the outdoors early does not necessarily mean they'll become avid backpackers later on, so don't be disappointed if they eventually lose interest.

If you want your children to grow to love hiking and the outdoors as much as you do, don't push too hard. If you try to do too much, they will only have unpleasant memories. Be content just to get out on the trail, instead of setting big mileage goals.

Chapter Fourteen

Long-distance Hiking

*I go forth to make new demands on life.
I wish to begin this summer well; to do
something in it worthy of it and me; to
transcend my daily routine and that of
my townsmen . . . I pray that the life of
this spring and summer may ever lie
fair in my memory. May I dare as
I have never done! May I persevere
as I have never done!*

—HENRY DAVID THOREAU

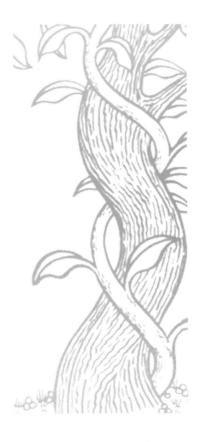

T horeau's words echo the sentiments of many people who set out each year intending to follow the white blazes along the Trail's entire length, be it from Georgia to Maine as most do, or the reverse.

Those who set out on this goal are referred to as thru-hikers, and anyone who succeeds in completing the entire current A.T. in a single 12-month period is considered to have thru-hiked the Trail. Though the designation thru-hiker is the word of choice, the Appalachian Trail Conservancy prefers to use the term "2,000-miler."

The ATC defines a 2,000-miler as anyone who has hiked the entire trail between Springer Mountain in Georgia and Katahdin in Maine. The ATC's recognition policy gives equal recognition to thru-hikers and section-hikers and it recognizes blue-blazed trails or officially required roadwalks as possible options for the official, white-blazed route in the event of an emergency. As of 2004, the ATC had officially recognized 7,830 hike completions.

When considering recognition for hiking the entire A.T., the ATC cares only that you have hiked the entire length of the Trail, and not whether or not you carried a pack, hiked it in sections, or how long it took you. The recognition policy works on the honor system and the ATC assumes that you have made an honest effort to walk the Appalachian Trail.

If you are thinking about hiking the entire Appalachian Trail, you may want to consider a few things first. The estimated number of thru-hikers leaving Springer Mountain per year reached a thousand around 1993. That year, about 160 of those finished the Trail.

In 2003, the ATC Web site estimates that 1,750 intended thru-hikers left Springer Mountain. By Neel's Gap 30 miles to the north, 350 of those hikers had already left the Trail. Just 741 of the hikers made it as far as Harpers Ferry, West Virginia, with 391 of those making it all the way to Katahdin.

Of those who start out on a thru-hike, only about 20 percent make it the whole way in a single year; the other 80 percent leave their dreams by the wayside. This happens for a number of reasons, but mostly because the Trail turns out to be more than they bargained for. Unrealistic expectations are what cause most backpackers to walk away from their dream of an A.T. thru-hike.

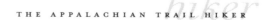

Just about any person has the physical ability to hike the entire A.T. It has been done by the young, the old, the physically challenged and everybody in between. But physical ability is not all it takes. It is easy to romanticize hiking the Appalachian Trail as an easy walk in the woods. It is almost never easy, and it is never just a walk in the woods.

WHAT IT TAKES TO BE A THRU-HIKER

I started with the intention of finishing," explained Doug Davis. "I think a lot of the quitters only committed themselves to giving it a try. As I went along I would try to imagine finishing [my thru-hike]. It was hard. I also tried to imagine not finishing. It was impossible."

Davis sums up the way most thru-hikers feel. It takes determination and goal orientation to finish the trail. Flexibility is the key.

Phil Hall said, "It takes determination, flexibility, and endurance. Without all three, you probably won't make it that far."

Steve Bekkala offers this question for prospective thru-hikers to ask themselves, "Can you think of a better way to spend your summer than hiking the A.T.? If the answer to that is yes, then you should be doing that instead."

Before you begin planning your hike, ask yourself these questions:

- Will completing the Trail be worth being wet/cold/hot day after day?
- Can I wear the same dirty clothes for days on end?
- Can I go without a bath, sometimes for as long as a week?
- Can I withstand the physical pain that often accompanies backpacking?
- Can I stand being away from my home/relationship for four to six months?
- Is the idea of thru-hiking the A.T. my all-consuming desire? Am I willing for it to be?
- Am I afraid of the outdoors—insects, animals, and sleeping outdoors night after night?

Some of these questions may seem trivial, but all of them point to reasons that people quit the trail. Obviously, severe physical injuries and emergencies at home also are a factor, but these have nothing to do with the determination, flexibility, and endurance it takes to hike the entire trail.

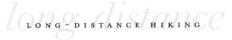

"Finishing the A.T. was all-important," said Sondra Davis, who hiked the Trail with her husband, Craig. "But enjoying it was reason enough."

What do we mean by flexibility, endurance, and determination? Consider this journal entry by Mac Wrightington penned at Vandeventer Shelter in Tennessee:

> First, the good news. Easy Ed [Ed Carlson] and I had a great time yesterday at Laurel Fork Shelter, and I slept fairly well despite reading in the register that a rat the size of a small dog resided there. I also had beautiful weather today.
>
> Now the bad [news]. The guidebook's description of the store at 321 [limited supplies] was the understatement of the century. For the next two days, it's corn flakes and water for breakfast, cookies for lunch, and pork and beans for dinner. Also, my feet, that gave me trouble yesterday, are now dead. No, wait a minute, if they were dead they wouldn't hurt this bad. My trusty Raichles have finally given out on me—causing bruises, blisters, and bleeding. Damascus is 32 miles away now, should be an interesting couple of days ahead.

Wrightington didn't enjoy his problems, but he also didn't think about quitting. Every hiker has at least one day like Wrightington's, usually many more. It's just something you have to keep in mind when you intend to hike for six months. Like six months in the "real" world, something is bound to go wrong occasionally.

WHY PEOPLE THRU-HIKE

There is no one reason that draws people to hike the entire Appalachian Trail. But there does seem to be a common denominator among thru-hikers: they are mostly at some period of change in their lives. A divorce, graduation from college or high school, retirement, marriage, and an anticipated change of careers are all typical times that hikers take to the A.T. to follow it from end to end.

HOW MUCH DOES IT COST TO HIKE?

How much do you want it to cost? A good rough estimate is $1 a mile, not including any equipment you may need. This is not going cheap, nor is it extravagant. If you are careful, the Appalachian Trail can be a very inexpensive six months. Your only real cost is food. Some hikers include the equipment they must purchase in the mile per dollar estimate and factor $1.50 to $2 a mile.

The ATC says that a thru-hike can cost from $1,000 to $5,000, not including equipment, with an average of about $3,000. The low end of the spectrum requires going without restaurant meals or motels, which few hikers prefer to pass up. Most people spend $1,000 to $2,000 on equipment.

You don't have to stay in hostels. You can conceivably camp instead of paying the few shelter fees. Other expenses include fuel for your stove. From there, what you spend is optional. Most hikers will splurge on restaurant meals when they go into town for food.

Other expenses might include:

- Laundry and detergent
- Entertainment (batteries for your walkman, movies, books, magazines, etc.)
- An occasional hotel/motel stay
- Replacement of gear (if you haven't already set aside a fund for emergencies)
- Doctor bills (also an emergency fund item)
- Miscellaneous items (batteries for your flashlight, stamps, stationery, etc.)

WHEN AND WHERE TO START

The majority of thru-hikers—about 70 percent—choose to start on Springer Mountain in Georgia and hike toward Katahdin in Maine. Another 20 percent start on Katahdin and head south, and the remaining 10 percent flip-flop or leap-frog. In the past several years, ATC has received approximately nine northbound "2,000-miler" completion reports for every one southbound report.

WEATHER

When using weather as a determinant in when and where to begin your hike, there are a number of things to keep in mind. The time of year, elevation, and latitude are the most important variables to consider. The most frequently overlooked one is elevation. For example, Blood Mountain, Georgia at 4,461 feet has colder temperatures and more snow than Harpers Ferry, West Virginia, which has an elevation of about 250 feet and is nearly a thousand trail miles to the north.

Because the Trail is often at high elevations, the potential for snow lasts into April and even early May in Georgia, the mid-Atlantic states, and much of New England, and until early June in New Hampshire and Maine.

The first snows of autumn usually occur in late September in Maine and New Hampshire and in October through the rest of New England. And though not as common, you can even find snow on the highest mountains of the South in the fall. In November any part of the Trail can receive snow.

In June, weather that is uncomfortably hot and humid for backpacking reaches from Georgia through Virginia, and into the mid-Atlantic states. July and August can be too hot for comfortable backpacking in much of the mid-Atlantic and South, although at elevations above 5,000 to 6,000 feet (North Carolina and Tennessee) the temperatures are often pleasant. High temperatures can linger sporadically into September in all areas along the A.T.

WHILE ON THE TRAIL

The following is suggested to keep your mind centered on a thru-hike:

- Be sure of your reasons for doing the Trail. Write them down somewhere, and check them occasionally to see if they are still valid.

- Take breaks every so often in hostels, trail towns, or even on the trail. These days of rest and pampering yourself are very important both physically and mentally.

- The entire A.T. is too long to set as a single goal. Split it up into sections or states, and celebrate each goal accomplished.

HIKING NORTH

For those who are considering hiking north along the A.T., most thru-hikers begin in mid-March to mid-April. It can take anywhere from five to seven months to complete the Trail, depending on your pace and how much time you take off along the way. Typically, though, if you start in March and finish in September, you can expect to start hiking with a lot more people—sometimes as many as 30 a day.

When beginning in March or April, you will experience some cold weather in the first two to three months. Snow and ice are not uncommon in Georgia and northward to Virginia. By the first of May, you should be seeing the first real signs of spring. Be prepared for deep snow in the high elevations of North Carolina, Tennessee, and as far north as the Mount Rogers area of Virginia.

Once you reach the mid-Atlantic states, you will begin to experience hot and humid weather during the summer months and by the time you reach New England, you will find the most enjoyable temperatures of the trip. But, if you are on the slow track, you can hit colder weather again in New Hampshire and Maine in the fall. The best thing about hiking northward is Katahdin. Climbing Katahdin at the end of your thru-hike makes for a very meaningful ending.

Northbounders must plan to reach Katahdin no later than mid-October, since Baxter State Park in Maine closes on October 15. If you are hiking north and you reach Harpers Ferry, West Virginia, after July 15, you should consider a

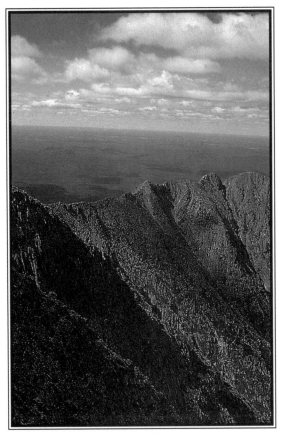

Looking north from atop Katahdin

"leapfrog" or a "flip-flop" hike (both discussed on page 217), unless you have covered the first thousand miles in two months or less. From Harpers Ferry, you still have almost 1,200 miles to go, and, once you reach the White Mountains, your daily mileage from there north through most of Maine will drop by a third. If you continue northward from Harpers Ferry after July 15, you may have to hike faster than you'd like, or face having to finish your hike another year.

Hikers who want to hike at a more relaxed pace or who find themselves falling behind schedule should plan on a flip-flop schedule (see page 217).

HIKING SOUTH

Some potential thru-hikers consider a southbound trip because they have to begin at a later date or because they are looking for solitude. Starting southward from Katahdin is more difficult but not impossible. Maine and New Hampshire are two of the toughest states on the Trail and starting in the north will give you a tougher breaking in period. Resupply points are farther apart so you have to carry a bit more food as well. According to the ATC, fewer than 400 people have reported finishing a southbound hike.

If you want to start from the north, Baxter State Park recommends that you begin no earlier than July 1. If you start before that time, you will add fierce black flies, possible snow, blowdowns, higher water at stream crossings, and muddy trail to your miseries. Your impact on the Trail will be a lot more damaging as well, as it is particularly fragile during the spring melt season.

Starting at Katahdin in July and ending at Springer in December, you will find that you hike mostly alone. As with northbound hikers, you will experience the humidty and heat of the mid-Atlantic but can look forward to fall foliage in Virginia.

Unfortunately, with fall foliage comes hunting season, and you will have to take the necessary precautions from Virginia southward. Finally, you might experience some cold weather, especially in higher elevations during November and December, and there is even the possibility of some snow.

ALTERNATE APPROACHES

Future thru-hikers who want to avoid crowded conditions the first few months of their hike may want to consider the different alternatives to starting in Georgia during thru-hiker season. There are advantages to an alternative hike, including starting on easier stretches of the A.T., during better weather conditions, or starting at times or places to avoid the crowds.

The easiest terrain on the A.T. is not at either end of the Trail, where thru-hikers normally start, but in the middle of the Trail (from Shenandoah National Park in Virginia north through southern Pennsylvania). In both directions, the Trail gradually gets more difficult as you head north or south. If you want to break in your body more gently to the rigors of long-distance backpacking, avoid starting south of Virginia or in New Hampshire and Maine, the two most difficult states on the Trail.

Obviously, there are lots of options when it comes to hiking the Trail if you are not set on hiking it in one continuous hike. Hikes can be set up to take advantage of weather conditions, to find more solitude, to work around previous engagements, or to enjoy the different wildflower seasons.

FLIP-FLOPPING

Flip-flopping is essentially doing the Trail in two major sections. One of the most common ways to flip-flop is to hike north from the Southern A.T. terminus of Springer Mountain in Georgia to Harpers Ferry, West Virginia. Once there, the hiker would travel north to Katahdin, the northern terminus in Maine and hike south to Harpers Ferry.

For example, you might start at Springer during the second half of April and hike north, reaching Harpers Ferry in the middle of July; then flip to Katahdin. There you would hike south to Harpers Ferry and end your hike during the first half of November. Among the benefits of this type of hike would be starting at Springer without the crowds of hikers. You would minimize the chance of encountering snow during your entire hike and avoid the heat of the mid-Atlantic, as well. You also would not have to worry about reaching Katahdin before it closes on October 15. A flip-flop isn't necessarily a completely lonely experience either. There are northbounders who begin a later hike that you could travel with to Harpers Ferry, and southbounders to hike with as you head south to Harpers Ferry, but in much lesser numbers. You would also run into those same northbounders again as you hiked south. Finally, you have the opportunity to see the fall foliage of the mid-Atlantic as you finish up your hike.

Another option is to hike northward from Harpers Ferry to Katahdin and then flip back to Harpers Ferry and hike southward to Springer. Flip-flopping leaves a number of options, as you can see.

Some hikers set out to flip-flop the Trail because they feel it gives them more time, or because they cannot begin their hike until mid-summer and do not wish to hike entirely southbound. Beginning mid-summer around Harpers Ferry would allow you to hike with a good many of that year's northbounders. Harpers Ferry is often a beginning or ending place because it is near the halfway point on the A.T.; it is also the location of the ATC headquarters.

LEAPFROG

This type of hike would have you hike from Springer Mountain north to Harpers Ferry, southern New England north to Katahdin, and southern New England south to Harpers Ferry.

For example, the hike could begin at Springer during the second half of April. You would then hike north, reaching Harpers Ferry in the middle of July. From there, you would "leapfrog" to Great Barrington, Massachusetts, where you would hike north to Katahdin, finishing there in September. From Katahdin, you would return to Great Barrington and hike south to Harpers Ferry. The advantages to this type of hike would mean that you could start at Springer but still avoid the crowds. As in the flip-flop, you would have a minimal chance of snow or severe cold and also avoid the worst heat of the mid-Atlantic. You would hike in New England before the severe cold sets in but get to enjoy the fall colors there and in the mid-Atlantic. Finally, there would be no time pressure to reach Katahdin.

The major drawback to this type of hike is the additional logistics involved in getting you to different sections of the Trail.

2,000-MILERS (SECTION HIKING)

An alternative to thru-hiking the Appalachian Trail is to become a 2,000-miler. It is distinguished equally with thru-hiking by the ATC and is defined as anyone who completes the entire Appalachian Trail over a period of two or more years.

If you are unable to take five to seven months off for one long hike, you can break the Trail up into smaller sections to be hiked over the years. The ATC does not make a distinction between 2,000-milers and thru-hikers, and the completion of the Trail over many years is just as meaningful as hiking it in one long hike.

ADVANTAGES AND DISADVANTAGES TO ALTERNATE APPROACHES

If you leave Springer Mountain in March or early April, you will find viewpoints, shelters, and campsites crowded. The opportunities for privacy and solitude are limited by the number of people attempting a thru-hike. An average of more than 35 thru-hikers a day leave Springer between March 1 and April 1. Northbound thru-hikers create a large, moving group of people, the majority of whom are concentrated over a 300–400 mile stretch of the Trail.

Georgia is always the most crowded, but most of the hikers who quit their hike drop off the Trail in Georgia, usually during the first week or so. Also in the South, you will run into spring-break hikers. There are a number of colleges/universities and outdoors groups that feature hikes along the A.T. during the spring holidays. The treks are usually centered along the southern end of the Trail in March and April. Because of this, crowded conditions continue well into Virginia.

The main disadvantages of an alternative hike include psychological factors as well as problems with logistics (that is, getting to and from starting and ending points). While overcrowding on the Trail may detract from your experience, so can loneliness. Most people find they enjoy their hiking experience more if they have other hikers around with whom they can share both the hardships and the joys of backpacking. It can help, as well, to have other thru-hikers around who can encourage you to stick it out when you get bored or discouraged and feel like quitting.

It is worth noting here that family and friends at home can get you through the lonely times by offering their support through phone calls or surprise packages at maildrops. There weren't many times we wanted to quit, but it was often our family who helped pull us through. A box from my sister containing an Easter basket brightened an otherwise gloomy and wet day in Virginia, for example.

In most variations of the alternate thru-hike you will be ending at a point other than Katahdin, the northern terminus of the A.T. in Maine. Katahdin is a mile-high mountain, a monadnock that is hard to beat for a dramatic finish to a thru-hike. On a northbound hike, it can be a powerful draw to spur you on. But, climbing Katahdin is an awesome event whether it is hiked first, last, or in between. And, if you climb Katahdin earlier in your journey, you won't have to race the weather or rush to make Baxter State Park's October 15 deadline.

CONSIDERATIONS WHILE ON THE TRAIL

HIKE YOUR OWN HIKE

A hiker who is not following one of the two standard thru-hikes—northbound or southbound—is likely to meet up with hikers who diss their thru-hike and treat them as if they are "wrong" for going about it in anyway but a straight-through hike. Some hikers find that this peer pressure detracts from their ability to enjoy their experience. Others miss the continuity and simplicity of a straight-through trek. If you need to experience a "through" hike as in starting at one end and ending at the other, it is best to do just that.

Lots of hikers, though, find they have to scramble their hike once they get started. We started the Appalachian Trail with every intention of beginning in Georgia and hiking straight through to Maine. Shin splints in New Jersey forced us off the Trail for a week. When Frank had healed, we discovered that the group we had been hiking with was in Connecticut. We skipped up to Connecticut to hike with them and hiked as far as Vermont before we realized that we didn't really want to leave the missing piece until the end of our hike. Hitching back to Connecticut, we hiked southward back to New Jersey before returning to Vermont and completing our hike. Our odd little hike didn't detract from our experience and in some ways broadened it.

While some additional logistical planning and expense might be required to get to the second (or third or fourth, etc.) leg of your journey, a number of reasons can lead to a sectioned hike. Those who plan to leave the A.T. for a brief hiatus—graduation, wedding etc.—may find that this type of hike fits conveniently into their travel plans.

Blue-blazing

Before you begin your thru-hike, you should make an important decision: just what is the goal you are pursuing? Is it to hike the entire Appalachian Trail, or is it merely to spend several months hiking in the Appalachians? You should ask yourself this question because opportunities will arise to cut off sections of the Trail to make it shorter, easier, or to provide easier access to shelters and towns.

The term for taking these shortcuts is blue-blazing. The name comes from the fact that most of the trails you will intersect are marked with blue blazes instead of the A.T.'s familiar white blazes. Hikers who stick to the white-blazed trail think of themselves as purists because they are staying true to their goal of hiking the entire trail.

If you decide ahead of time how "pure" you want your hike to be, you will have less trouble later. We discovered that once you begin to blue-blaze it is harder not to do so again.

The ATC does not take an official stand on blue-blazing. Most hikers consider it acceptable to take a loop trail to a shelter and come back to the white-blazed trail by the other side of the loop. This only cuts off 0.1 or 0.2 miles, and is common practice.

An example of an extreme case of blue-blazing would be taking the Tuckerman Ravine trail down from Mount Washington in New Hampshire to cut off the 12.9-mile hike across the Northern Presidential Range in less than 5 miles of downhill trail. So you can see that making a distinction before you leave home will help you choose which trail to follow once you're hiking. The ATC will have expected you to hike the entire white-blazed Trail unless blue-blazed sections were used for emergency situations such as a flood, a forest fire, or an impending storm on an exposed, high-elevation stretch. Because the ATC works on the honor system, it will be on your conscience as to how much you blue-blaze.

Whatever choice you make for yourself, remember that you are hiking for your own reasons and to meet your own goals. Allow others the same courtesy. Try not to view another's hiking style as wrong; it is only different.

Trail Etiquette

The success of a thru-hiker's journey depends heavily on Trail towns and the services they provide. Likewise, the continued success of the A.T. and the ATC depends on the support of the people who live near the Trail. Nothing can turn a person or town against backpacking and the A.T. quicker than an ill-behaved hiker. In recent years, some businesses have closed their doors or reduced the services they offer because of problems with hikers. In town, consider yourself a walking, talking billboard for backpacking and the Appalachian Trail.

The Appalachian Long-Distance Hikers Association (ALDHA) and ATC are working to reverse this unfortunate trend, and you can make a difference as well. When in town, remember you are a guest, even though you may be pumping money into the local economy. Be courteous to those who make their living there, and remember your conduct will have a bearing on how well the next hiker is treated. Always, always follow rules and regulations posted at hostels. Just because you are living in the woods temporarily, doesn't mean you have license to act like an animal.

If you would like to give back what was freely given to you while you stayed in Trail towns, volunteer your time, effort, or money to the services and people who supported you. Consider organizing or participating in a work trip. Every year, the ALDHA sponsors at least two work trips to Trail establishments; this helps keep services available, and it lets facilities know that their goodwill is appreciated by the hiking community.

Money

You will probably want to take some form of money with you along the Trail to occasionally splurge at an all-you-can-eat buffet or stay at a nice hotel. However, hiking with up to $1,000 in cash is a bad way to test your trust in your fellow humans. Most hikers choose the safety and convenience of either carrying traveler's checks or using a credit or debit card.

Traveler's checks can be cashed almost anywhere. We haven't heard of any store along the A.T., no matter how small or out-of-the-way, that wouldn't cash a traveler's check. By buying the checks in varying denominations, you can assure that you won't be caught carrying a large amount of cash at any one time. For added peace of mind, and to help stay on budget, it is a good idea to split your traveler's checks up into two or three envelopes to send to some of your maildrops.

Automated teller machines have made their way to most of the towns along the Trail and have become a reliable way to receive money as well. Through credit cards or bank cards that are part of a nationwide network, hikers can obtain money in an emergency or as part of a scheduled withdrawal. Most grocery stores are equipped to take debit as well as credit cards.

Whether you intend to use your credit card for cash withdrawals or not, plan to bring it along. A major credit card can be a lifesaver if equipment breaks or medical problems arise. Phone cards are helpful in reaching family and friends from the A.T. and can be used to contact equipment manufacturers in an emergency.

INSURANCE

Setting out to hike the length of the A.T. without medical insurance is folly at best, though many hikers take this route. The best option for most hikers is to stick with the insurance available from your last employer. Thanks to a 1986 act of Congress, known by the acronym COBRA, certain former employees, retirees, spouses, and dependent children have the right to temporary continuation of health coverage at group rates. A couple of caveats are in order, however. This coverage is available only in specific instances. Group health coverage for COBRA participants is usually more costly than health coverage for active employees, since usually the employer formerly paid a part of the premium. But, coverage through the COBRA provision is ordinarily less expensive than buying individual health coverage.

If you do not qualify to extend a policy through COBRA, comparably low-cost, short-term medical insurance is available through most companies. The short-term policies are designed for people between jobs and typically last no longer than six months. This type of policy is nonrenewable but allows enough coverage for the duration of an A.T. thru-hike. As with any policy, the higher the deductible, the lower the premiums will be.

MAILDROPS

The majority of hikers buy their food along the way, but some mail their food ahead. This requires planning before you hit the trail, so packages arrive just ahead of your need for them. Using a number of maildrops for food or any other essential (e.g., traveler's checks) will mean that you will have to schedule your hike around getting to town when the post office, hostel, or store is open. Space your pick-ups about 70 to 100 miles apart if used as your primary food source;

150 to 200 miles apart or more should be sufficient if you don't use them as your only source of food.

When you send a package, here is how you should address it:

Your name c/o General Delivery
City, state zip code
Return address
Please hold for [northbound/southbound] A.T. thru-hiker.
Date you expect to pick up package

Letters and packages marked "Hold for northbound (or southbound) A.T. thru-hiker" help ensure (but not guarantee) that the post office will hold them much longer than customary (usually 30 days, though occasionally a post office may return them sooner). Post offices, hostels, or stores frequented by hikers generally refrain from returning packages until that year's group of hikers stops coming by, though with increasing numbers of hikers, post offices may no longer be able to hold packages as long as they have in the past.

Zip codes for post offices near the A.T. and distances from the Trail to the post office are given in the annually updated *Data Book* published by the Appalachian Trail Conservancy. Other resources for planning your maildrops are *The Appalachian Trail Workbook for Planning Thru-hikes* and the *Appalachian Trail Thru-hiker's Companion*, which are also published by the ATC.

As nice as receiving mail can be, remember that maildrops can also be a nuisance. If you come into a town after noon on Saturday, you will probably have to wait until Monday morning for mail. If the maildrop is not essential, you can send or leave a forwarding card and let the mail catch up to you later.

It is always a good idea to fill out a forwarding card at any post office you use, even if you're not expecting additional mail. Forward your mail ahead to a post office you expect to reach in two or three weeks or to your home address. To forward a package, you are required to fill out Form 3575. (You cannot forward a package by a telephone request.) If you plan to receive jointly addressed packages, list both names on the form. Priority Mail and first-class mail can be forwarded at no additional cost; a third-class package cannot be forwarded. A package cannot be forwarded after it is opened.

Post offices are not obligated to provide mailing tape free of charge, but some post offices offer it for sale. It's a good idea to include mailing tape, labels, and magic markers in your food packages or your send-ahead box.

The post office cannot accept a FedEx or UPS package so make sure that you inform whoever is sending your packages to send them by U.S. mail. Post offices now accept credit cards and ATM cards. On ATM purchases, you can get up to $50 cash back, provided the post office has the cash on hand. (Small post offices may not have this much cash on hand, especially in the morning.)

Even if you don't intend to send your food ahead, you should still plan on a few maildrops. Sending film, guidebooks and maps, Sno-Seal, seam sealer, contact-lens solution, or other hard-to-get items are some good uses for a maildrop.

"One of the most helpful things I did for myself about a third of the way through the trip was to have a box that I continually sent ahead of myself," said Rob White. "I used the box to send excess equipment up the Trail for me. And when I decided to get rid of my tent and use the tarp, I sent the tent about a week ahead before I sent it home."

Friends and family can also be given a list of post offices where you plan to check for mail; this usually produces a variety of letters and packages, making all your planning worthwhile.

HIKING PARTNERS

Many people who wish to hike the entire length of the A.T. do not wish to do so alone. Is it possible to find an appropriate partner? Possible, yes. Easy, no.

ATC members may submit an advertisement for a partner in the Public Notices section of the *Appalachian Trailway News* at no charge. There are a number of A.T.-related Web-based forums and discussion groups where you can post messages expressing interest in a hiking partner. In addition, discussion groups for A.T. hikers interested in thru-hiking for a particular year usually form a Yahoo listserve group with that online service.

While finding a partner through an ad usually works out, the truth is that these types of partnerships rarely last long on the trail. But, if finding a partner through an ad will help to get you out on the trail it might be worth the effort. Hiking with a partner can help you gain confidence in your own abilities until you are confident enough to either hike on your own or hook up with a new partner.

If you don't want to find a partner through an ad, you can easily find people to hike with by starting your thru-hike during peak hiking season—March 1 through mid-April. During this time there are so many potential thru-hikers starting out that whether you like it or not, you'll be sharing shelters and trail nearly all the way to Maine.

Some more advice for those hiking with partners or spouses:

"Undertaking a thru-hike with another person is a more intense experience than marriage," said Bill O'Brien, who hiked with Andrew Sam. "At least in marriage, you each presumably go off to work at different jobs. On a thru-hike, you're together always, day and night."

Andrew Sam agreed, adding, "Don't feel obligated to hike together during the day. Meet up at lunch and at a campsite. Above all, be flexible."

Some couples prefer to split up during the day while others don't mind the constant companionship. Cal and Mary Batchelder recommend, "If you wish to hike right behind each other (but not too close), hike at the slowest hiker's pace." Frank and I thru-hiked this way, successfully, and continue to do so whenever we backpack with our daughter.

HOSTELS

A hostel can be as simple as the floor of a church or barn, or it may offer as much as a hot shower, warm bed, laundry facilities, and food. Hostels range in price from free (although a donation is always appreciated) to $20 or more a night. All offer a deal to hikers that should be used but not taken advantage of. It is a good idea to limit your stay to a night or two (unless it's an emergency), if the hostel is run by volunteers on a donation basis.

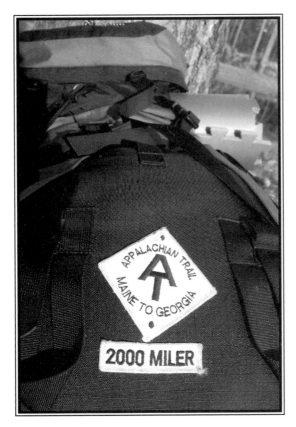

Old-style ATC patch with 2,000-miler chevron beneath

If you intend to stay in hostels during a thru-hike, count on leaving at least a small donation (even if they don't ask for it). Some hostels will let you work off your stay, but all appreciate a helping hand even if you're paying. If the hostel is a business, you need only be courteous and may stay as long as you are willing to pay for a room or bed; but if it is run by volunteers, help out. Prove that thru-hikers are not the socially irresponsible crowd a lot of people think they are. Try to clean up behind other hikers as well as yourself. A good attitude goes a long way toward improving relations along the Appalachian Trail.

A current listing of hostels can be found in *The Appalachian Trail Thruhiker's Companion.*

Huts

The hut system run by the Appalachian Mountain Club (AMC) is another area where thru-hikers need to be on their best behavior. The huts were built and run long before thru-hikers existed, and the AMC makes most of its money in the Whites not from thru-hikers but from hikers who come to hike hut-to-hut. More information on the A.M.C.'s hut system is found in the chapter on hike preparation.

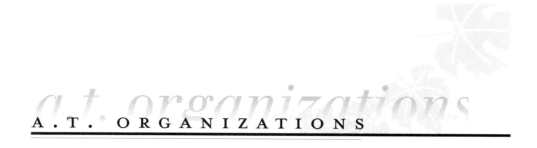

A.T. ORGANIZATIONS

APPALACHIAN LONG-DISTANCE HIKERS ASSOCIATION

ALDHA was the first organization of long-distance hikers in the United States (and led to the creation of an ALDHA West). Although its focus is on the A.T., ALDHA also promotes long-distance trails around the world. For those interested in hiking the A.T., ALDHA is a great organization to join. Each year, ALDHA hosts The Gathering of Long-Distance Hikers (it is usually just called "The Gathering"). The Gathering is not limited to those who have hiked the Appalachian and other trails. Future hikers and trail helpers also attend.

For $17 per person or $27 per couple, hikers are treated to a Columbus Day weekend of workshops (including an extensive workshop on preparing for an A.T. hike), slideshows, music and dancing, and the camaraderie of hikers and hiker friends. A campsite is included in the fee, but meals are extra. The fee includes a $7 annual ALDHA membership ($150 lifetime membership). ALDHA members receive a quarterly newsletter, *The Long-Distance Hiker*, and a membership directory. For more information, contact:

ALDHA
10 Benning Street
PMB 224
West Lebanon, NH 03784
www.aldha.org

THE APPALACHIAN TRAIL CONSERVANCY

Hikers dreaming of hiking all or part of the Appalachian Trail are advised to join the Appalachian Trail Conservancy. When you join or renew your ATC membership, you'll receive:

1) A year's subscription to the *Appalachian Trailway News*, ATC's member magazine devoted to helping you explore and enjoy the Trail.

2) Discounts of up to 20 percent on ATC publications and merchandise, including its maps and books—the trusted guides found in so many backpacks on the A.T.

3) An annual decal and membership card and, for first-year new members, an embroidered, members-only patch.

4) The right to vote on the election of ATC's volunteer board of managers and Conservancy resolutions at their biennial membership gatherings—a week-long event that combines business with the pleasure of recreational workshops, family entertainment, and, of course, hikes on the Trail.

5) ATC's Life Membership Endowment Fund. As an ATC life member, discounts on all ATC merchandise and your subscription to the *Appalachian Trailway News* last your lifetime. You'll receive a new ATC decal each year, a special lifetime membership card and special patch, and be listed in ATC's Annual Report in the year you become a life member. Most of all, you'll know that your gift will be placed in the ATC's life membership endowment fund, providing legacy funding to ATC's programs to build and protect the A.T.

Memberships in the ATC range from $25 for a "Caretaker"—an A.T. maintaining club member, senior (65 and older), or student—to $900 for life membership for a couple.

THE AFTERLIFE

Once you have completed your thru-hike or section-hike of the A.T., you can send in a report form that is your application for 2,000 Miler status. The forms can be found on the Trail at Katahdin Stream Campground in Baxter State Park, Maine, and at the Walasi-Yi Center in Neels Gap, Georgia, and at Amicalola Falls State Park in Georgia. The forms are online at **www.appalachiantrail.org/hike/pdfs/2Kmiler03.pdf.** You can also pick up a form from ATC Headquarters at 799 Washington Street in Harpers Ferry, WV 25425, order one by calling (304) 535-6331, or by e-mailing the ATC Information Center (info@appalachiantrail.org).

Two-thousand-milers who submit a completed application to ATC will receive a certificate of recognition from the Conservancy and a 2,000-miler rocker for an A.T. patch (the conference works with volunteer help to process the applications as quickly as they can, but please allow 12 weeks to receive your have their name added to the ATC's official database of 2,000-milers, and receive a one-time listing in the *Appalachian Trailway News* (usually in the May/June edition following application submission).

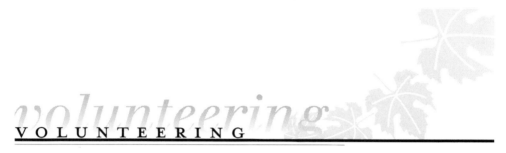

VOLUNTEERING

I f you haven't done so already, a great way to give back to the A.T. is by volunteering. The Trail was built through volunteer labor and volunteers continue to maintain the Appalachian Trail today. From simple trail maintenance to relocations and even building shelters and privies, volunteers in trail clubs and work crews keep the Trail in existence.

Although the A.T. is a National Scenic Trail, which is managed under the auspices of the National Park Service, it is maintained by volunteers who do most of the work necessary to administer this 2,160-mile-long footpath. More than 4,000 volunteers contribute their time and talent each year to keep the trailway open so that the millions of people who use it each year can continue to enjoy it. There are a number of ways you can volunteer.

Join a local maintaining club. There are more than 30 different clubs active along the length of the A.T. Throughout the year, the volunteers in these clubs do the essential work that keeps the Trail cleared and in good repair. By clearing brush, removing blowdowns, constructing shelters and bridges, monitoring rare and endangered species along with a host of other activities, the clubs preserve the integrity of the footpath and the corridor that surrounds it.

To join forces with these trail caretakers, contact the club nearest you (see page 237). Maintaining clubs welcome those who want to work to care for the footpath, as well as those with administrative, clerical, and management or professional skills.

Another option is to join a trail crew. There are times when the trail work required calls for more than casual maintenance. In this case, special expertise as well as extra muscle power is needed. When this is the case, trail clubs will contact the regional office and request a trail crew. If approved, a crew will be sent that is managed by professionals with volunteers to do the work. If you can devote at least five days at a time, and don't mind putting in a little hard labor, you will be taught the necessary skills to build a piece of trail or rehabilitate an eroded section. The end product is often priceless in the amount of satisfaction achieved by producing something enjoyed by thousands of hikers. If you wish to apply, a brochure and application are available through both the Conservancy and its Web site. You may also request information by emailing crews@appalachiantrail.org.

The ATC's central office in historic Harpers Ferry, West Virginia, supports the work of all the Trail's management and its protection programs. While the ATC headquarters is staffed by professionals, it is the volunteers who help keep the offices running. The ATC welcomes you to join the regular local volunteers who come by the Conservancy once a week or once a month. If you live too far for the occasional trip, you might want to consider volunteering for a week, a month, or longer. The ATC is willing to provide lodging for long-term volunteers. They usually have plenty of projects for walk-in (or even hike-in) volunteers. Whether you would like to stuff envelopes, answer information questions, or apply any special talents and skills you might have to helping the land trust or other programs, the ATC can always use your help.

As a special incentive, a limited-edition T-shirt is awarded to volunteers who work 40 hours, and volunteers can also receive a special discount on ATC merchandise. The Conservancy also offers free lodging at the nearby Bears Den hostel (a vehicle is required for the 25-mile commute). And, alternate arrangements can be made for long-term volunteers who lack transportation. If space is available, volunteers can use one of the conservancy's two apartments.

ATC's Land Trust has benefited enormously from the efforts of long-term volunteers. Recent projects spearheaded by long-term volunteers include a multi-year mapping program, a demographic study, and a symposia. If you are interested in learning how you can volunteer with the ATC Land Trust, contact landtrust@appalachiantrail.org.

Proper planning is essential for any long-distance hike on the Appalachian Trail, but don't take it too far. "There's such a thing as doing too much research," offers thru-hiker Joe Cook. "If you know what's around every curve in the Trail, you have missed out on one of the most exciting parts of a thru-hike. Rely some on your own instincts and experience to guide you."

Appendixes

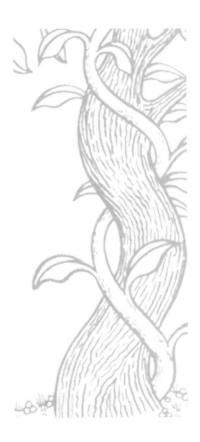

EQUIPMENT CHECKLISTS

Equipment for a Day Hike

(This list assumes you are already wearing comfortable clothes and good walking shoes.)

Day pack or fanny pack

One-liter (minimum) canteen

Rain gear

Food for the day

Lighter or waterproof matches

First aid (bandages, moleskin)

Toilet paper, trowel

Map and/or guidebook*

Camera and film*

Binoculars*

Gloves and knit cap+

Extra shirt+

Bandana*

Equipment for an Overnight Hike

Light- or mediumweight hiking boots

Internal- or external-frame pack

Sleeping bag

Sleeping pad

Tent/tarp and groundcloth

Lighter and/or waterproof matches

Stove and fuel

Cooking pot and eating utensils

Knife (pocket)

Water purifier, such as filter (or plan to boil your water)

More than adequate food for length of hike

Spices*

One-liter (minimum) canteen

Drinking cup

Rain gear including pack cover

Gaiters*

One pair of shorts

One pair of loose fitting, long pants+

One to two short-sleeve shirts

One long-sleeve shirt or sweater

Knit cap

Two pairs liner socks

Two pairs socks

One or more bandanas

Long johns+

Parka (down or synthetic fill)+

Underwear (2 pair)*

Toilet paper, trowel

Biodegradable soap and washcloth

Deodorant*

Toothbrush and toothpaste

Shaving kit*

Nylon cord (at least 25 feet)

Maps, guidebooks, or *Data Book*

Compass*

Flashlight with new batteries

Watch or clock*

Sunglasses*

First-aid kit (including moleskin)

Space blanket

Swimsuit and towel*

Extra shoes*

Repair equipment (for pack, tent, and stove)*

Camera and film*

Radio with headphones*

Insect repellent+

Sunscreen/lotion+

Hiking stick*

Additional Equipment for Longer Hikes

Repair equipment for pack, tent, stove, and clothes

Trash bag (a small one for your own trash)

Long-sleeve shirt or sweater

Long johns

Film mailers*

*The Appalachian Trail Companion**

Reading material*

Journal*

*Optional

+Seasonal

APPENDIX TWO

BOOKS ABOUT THE APPALACHIAN TRAIL

The following books are available from the Appalachian Trail Conservancy, P. O. Box 807, Harpers Ferry, WV 25425, as well as outdoor retailers and bookstores.

2,000 Miles on the Appalachian Trail, by Don Fortunato. An illustrated account of an early 1980s thru-hike of the A.T.

A.T. Design, Construction, and Maintenance, by William Burchard, Bob Proudman, and the ATC Regional Staff. 2000. The definitive guide to Trail building and maintenance on the East Coast.

Appalachian National Scenic Trail: A Time to Be Bold, by Charles H. W. Foster. 1987. A history of the Trail and its public protection.

The Appalachian Trail: Calling Me Back to the Hills, by Earl Shaffer and Bart Smith. 2002. 128 pages of prose and poetry by the first-ever A.T. thru-hiker, written after his third thru-hike in 1998 at the age of 79. Shaffer's words are accompanied by Smith's A.T. photos.

The Appalachian Trail Companion, edited by the Appalachian Long-Distance Hikers Association. An annually updated companion to the *Data Book* for long-distance hikers. This on-trail guide gives details on what services are available along the Trail, and more.

Appalachian Trail Data Book, compiled by Daniel D. Chazin. An annually updated guide featuring mileages between features and facilities on the Trail.

Appalachian Trail Fun Book, by Frank and Victoria Logue. 1993. A 72-page coloring and activity book designed to introduce four- to nine-year-olds to the Appalachian Trail.

Appalachian Trail Guides, published by the Appalachian Trail Conservancy. The eleven official Trail guides are published by the ATC or its member clubs and are updated every two to three years in most cases. Each guide is a pocket-sized book detailing a section of the Trail and comes with up to 12 topographic maps of that section. All guides are sold in a waterproof plastic pouch.

Maine	*New Hampshire/Vermont*	*Massachusetts/Connecticut*
New York/New Jersey	*Pennsylvania*	*Maryland/Northern Virginia*
Shenandoah National Park	*Central Virginia*	*Southwest Virginia*
Tennessee/North Carolina	*(Includes the Great Smoky Mountains National Park)*	
North Carolina/Georgia	*(Includes the Great Smoky Mountains National Park)*	

Appalachian Trail in Bits and Pieces, by Mary Sands. 1993. A recount of 16 years of hikes covering the entire A.T. with 100 Girl Scout companions.

Appalachian Trail on My Mind, by Globe Pequot Press. 2002. A 96-page compilation of words and pictures on the Appalachian Trail.

The Appalachian Trail Reader, by David Emblidge. 1997. A 1990s compendium of previously published articles and excerpts from books.

Appalachian Trail Workbook for Planning Thru-Hikes, by Chris Whalen. 1991. A rip-out-the-pages workbook of checklists, maildrops, etc.

As Far as the Eye Can See, by David Brill. 1990. A well-written and reflective account of a 1978 thru-hiker.

Backpacker magazine's Guide to the Appalachian Trail, by Jim Chase. 1989. A history of the Trail combined with anecdotes.

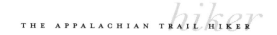

The Best of the Appalachian Trail: Day Hikes, by Victoria and Frank Logue and Leonard Adkins. 2004. With 150 hikes in all fourteen Trail states, this book guides hikers to the best day hikes on the Appalachian Trail. There is an overview of the hike, point-by-point description, and complete trailhead directions for each of the hikes, which are also rated for difficulty and given an approximate length of time the hike will take.

The Best of the Appalachian Trail: Overnight Hikes, by Victoria and Frank Logue and Leonard Adkins. 2004. A companion to the day-hikes book above, this guide includes more than 70 overnight hikes along the Trail. Each hike is rated for difficulty from easy to strenuous.

Blind Courage: Journey of Faith, by Bill Irwin and David McCasland. 1992. A stirring account of a blind hiker's 1990 thru-hike of the A.T. with his dog, Orient.

Breaking Trail in the Central Appalachians, by David Bates. 1987. The history of the Potomac Appalachian Trail Club.

Geology of the Appalachian Trail in Pennsylvania, by J. Peter Wilshusen. 1983. The geologic history of Pennsylvania's 230 miles of Trail.

Hiking the Triple Crown: Appalachian Trail—Pacific Crest Trail—Continental Divide Trail. How to Hike America's Longest Trails, by Karen Berger. 2001. A how-to guide to America's three great trails from a hiker who has done the Triple Crown herself and knows how to convey the information in a direct and highly readable style.

A Journey North: One Woman's Story of Hiking the Appalachian Trail, by Adrienne Hall. 2000. A non-romantic account of an A.T. thru-hike that shares all the woes from sore muscles to bugs and more.

Katahdin with Love: An Inspirational Journey, by Madelaine Cornelius. 1990. A couple's story of their A.T. thru-hike begun after the death of their son.

Long Distance Hiking: Lessons from the Appalachian Trail, by Roland Mueser. 1997. Mueser surveyed 136 A.T. thru-hikers to compile this how-to guide to long-distance hiking on the A.T.

Mountain Adventure: Exploring the Appalachian Trail, by Ron Fisher, photographs by Sam Abell. 1989. Published by the National Geographic Society, this book charts a south-to-north thru-hike by talking to hikers, maintainers, and people who live near the Trail.

The New Appalchian Trail, by Edward B. Garvey. 1997. This is the latest book by the author of the popular but now out-of-print *Appalachian Hiker* and *Appalachian Hiker II.* It mixes experiences from Ed's five-month-long A.T. hike, which he took at the age of 75, with information on gear, Trail etiquette, and more.

On the Beaten Path: An Appalachian Pilgrimage, by Robert Alden Rubin. 2000. This well-written tale gives an honest account of an A.T. thru-hike that is well worth the read.

A Season on the Appalachian Trail, by Lynn Setzer. 1997. This book follows hikers from

Georgia to Maine as the writer interviews thru-hikers at a number of key locations to provide a window on the A.T. experience.

A Time to Walk: Life Lesson Learned on the Appalachian Trail, by Jay Platt. 2000. Platt distills ten life lessons from his 1998 A.T. thru-hike and illustrates the lessons with stories from his hike.

Underfoot: A Geologic Guide to the Appalachian Trail, by V. Collins Chew. Revised 1993. A guide to the geology of the entire A.T., including a history of the formation of the Appalachian Mountain chain.

A Walk for Sunshine: A 2,160-mile Expedition for Charity on the Appalachian Trail, by Jeff Alt. 2000. Alt's book tells of his thru-hike to raise money for the Sunshine Home, which cares for 850 developmentally disabled residents.

A Walk in the Woods: Rediscovering America on the Appalachian Trail, by Bill Bryson. 1998. A humorous account of an A.T. hike (though not a thru-hike) that is a good source of laughs, but a questionable-at-best source of reliable information on the Trail. This book was a New York Times Bestseller.

Walking the Appalachian Trail, by Larry Luxenberg. 1994. Thru-hiker Larry Luxenburg interviewed dozens of A.T. hikers to capture the thru-hiking experience.

Walking Home, A Woman's Pilgrimage on the Appalachian Trail, by Kelly Winters. 1991. A woman's experience of empowerment in and through a late-1990s thru-hike.

Walking North, by Mic Lowther. 2000. A well-written account of a family's A.T. thru-hike in the 1970s.

Walkin' on the Happy Side of Misery: A Slice of Life on the Appalachian Trail, by Junius R. Tate. 2001. The story of three 1990s A.T. thru-hikes, with more than a touch of good humor.

Walking with Spring, by Earl Shaffer. 1987. Shaffer's story of his 1948 thru-hike. Shaffer was the first to hike the entire Appalachian Trail in a single year.

White Blaze Fever, by Bill Schuette. 2003. The story of one retirees' thru-hike, this book also contains more than one hundred hiker tips to assist future generations of thru-hikers.

Wildflowers of the Appalachian Trail, by Leonard M. Adkins with photos by Joe and Monica Cook. 1999. This absolutely beautiful book is a great reference source for where to find and how to identify the many wildflowers along the Appalachian Trail.

A Woman's Journey, by Cindy Ross. 1982. The personal story of Ross's two-year, 2,100-mile journey on the A.T. in the late 1970s, illustrated with her charcoal sketches.

TRAIL MAINTENANCE CLUBS

The Appalachian Trail owes its existence to the hiking clubs, which are charged with its maintenance. These clubs are responsible not only for the maintenance of the footpath but also for relocating the Trail, managing its surrounding lands, helping with land-acquisition negotiations, compiling and updating guidebook and map information, working with Trail communities on both problems and special events, and recruiting and training new maintainers.

The A.T. is maintained and protected by clubs and organizations along its length. If you are interested in local hikes or other activities in your area, check out the clubs and Trail organizations near you.

Addresses appear for those with permanent offices or post office boxes. Occasionally these do change; in this case, please contact ATC headquarters for the address of the current club president or other appropriate officer (P. O. Box 807, Harpers Ferry, West Virginia 25425, or **www.appalachiantrail.org**).

GEORGIA, NORTH CAROLINA, AND TENNESSEe

Georgia Appalachian Trail Club
P. O. Box 654, Atlanta, GA 30301
Voice mailbox: (404) 634-6495
www.georgia-atclub.org
Springer Mountain to Bly Gap, NC

Nantahala Hiking Club
173 Carl Slagle Road
Franklin, NC 28734
www.maconweb.com/nhc
Bly Gap, NC to Wesser, NC

Smoky Mountains Hiking Club
P. O. Box 1454
Knoxville, TN 37901
www.esper.com/smhc
Wesser, NC to Davenport Gap

Carolina Mountain Club
P. O. Box 68
Asheville, NC 28802
www.carolinamtnclub.com
Davenport Gap to Spivey Gap, NC

Tennessee Eastman Hiking Club
P. O. Box 511
Kingsport, TN 37662
www.tehcc.org
Spivey Gap, NC to Damascus, VA

VIRGINIA, WEST VIRGINIA, AND MARYLAND

Mount Rogers Appalachian Trail Club
24198 Green Spring Road
Abingdon, VA 24211-5320
www.geocities.com/Yosemite/Geyser/253
Damascus, VA to VA 670

Piedmont Appalachian Trail Hikers
P. O. Box 4423
Greensboro, NC 27404
www.path-at.org
VA 670 to VA 623; VA 615 to VA 612

Outdoor Club of Virginia Tech
P. O. Box 538
Blacksburg, VA 24063
www.fbox.vt.edu/org/outdoor
VA 623 to VA 615; VA 612 to VA 611; US
460 to Pine Swamp Branch Shelter

Roanoke Appalachian Trail Club
P. O. Box 12282
Roanoke, VA 24024
www.ratc.org
VA 611 to US 460; Pine Swamp Branch
Shelter to Black Horse Gap

Natural Bridge Appalachian Trail Club
P. O. Box 3012
Lynchburg, VA 24503
www.nbatc.org
Black Horse Gap to Tye River

Tidewater Appalachian Trail Club
P. O. Box 8246
Norfolk, VA 23503
www.tidewateratc.org
Tye River to Reeds Gap

Old Dominion Appalachian Trail Club
P. O. Box 25283
Richmond, VA 23260
www.odatc.org
Reeds Gap to Rockfish Gap

Potomac Appalachian Trail Club
118 Park Street SE
Vienna, VA 22180
(703) 242-0693
www.patc.net
Rockfish Gap, VA to Pine Grove Furnace
State Park, PA

PATC Local Chapters
Charlottesville Chapter
John Shannon, (434) 293-2953

Southern Shenandoah Valley Chapter
Michael Seth, (540) 438-1301

Northern Shenandoah Valley Chapter
Lee Sheaffer, (540) 955-0736
thumpers@visuallink.com

West Virginia Chapter
Judy Smoot, (540) 667-2036
wvpatc@hotmail.com;
www.patc-wv.org

North Chapter
Pete Brown, (410) 343-1140
northchapter@patc.net
www.patc.net/chapters/north

PENNSYLVANIA
The Potomac Appalachian Trail Club also
maintains the A.T. in Pennsylvania, from
the PA–Maryland state line to Pine Grove
Furnace State Park.

Keystone Trails Association
P. O. Box 129
Confluence, PA 15424
www.kta–hike.org
KTA is the umbrella organization for clubs
throughout Pennsylvania, some of which
maintain the A.T.

Mountain Club of Maryland
7923 Galloping Circle
Baltimore, MD 21244-1254
(410) 377-6266
www.mcomd.org
Pine Grove Furnace State Park, PA to Center Point Knob; Darlington Trail to Susquehanna River

Cumberland Valley Appalachian Trail Club
P. O. Box 395
Boiling Springs, PA 17007
www.geocities.com/cvatclub
Center Point Knob to Darlington Trail

York Hiking Club
2684 Forest Road
York, PA 17402
(717) 244-6769
www.angelfire.com/pa2/yorkhikingclub
  /index.html
Susquehanna River to PA 225

Susquehanna Appalachian Trail Club
P. O. Box 61001
Harrisburg, PA 17106-1001
www.libertynet.org/susqatc
PA 225 to Clarks Valley

Blue Mountain Eagle Climbing Club
P. O. Box 14982
Reading, PA 19612-4982
www.bmecc.org
Rausch Gap Shelter to Tri-County Corner;
Bake Oven Knob Road to Lehigh Furnace
Gap

Allentown Hiking Club
P. O. Box 1542
Allentown, PA 18105-1542
www.allentownhikingclub.org
Tri-County Corner to Bake Oven Knob Road

Philadelphia Trail Club
741 Golf Drive
Warrington, PA 18976
(215) 343-1695
www.m.zanger.tripod.com/index
Lehigh Furnace Gap to Little Gap

AMC-Delaware Valley Chapter
1180 Greenleaf Drive
Bethlehem, PA 18017-9319
www.amcdv.org
Little Gap to Wind Gap

Batona Hiking Club
6651 Eastwood Street
Philadelphia, PA 19149-2331
members.aol.com/Batona
Wind Gap to Fox Gap

Wilmington Trail Club
P. O. Box 1184
Wilmington, DE 19899
www.wilmingtontrailclub.org
Fox Gap to Delaware River

New Jersey and New York
New York-n-New Jersey Trail Conference
156 Ramapo Valley Road (Route 202)
Mahwah, NJ 07430-1199
(201) 512-9348
www.nynjtc.org
Delaware River to Connecticut–New York
border

**CONNECTICUT AND
MASSACHUSETTS**

AMC Connecticut Chapter
964 South Main Street
Great Barrington, MA 01230
(413) 528-6333
www.ct-amc.org
Connecticut–New York border to Sages
Ravine

AMC–Berkshire Chapter
964 South Main Street
Great Barrington, MA 01230
(413) 528-6333
www.amcberkshire.org
Sages Ravine to Vermont–Massachusetts
border

**VERMONT, NEW HAMPSHIRE, AND
MAINE**

Green Mountain Club
4711 Waterbury-Stowe Road
Waterbury Center, VT 05677
(802) 244-7037
www.greenmountainclub.org
Vermont–Massachusetts border to VT 12

Dartmouth Outing Club
P. O. Box 9
Hanover, NH 03755
(603) 646-2428
www.dartmouth.edu/~doc
VT 12 to Kinsman Notch, NH

Appalachian Mountain Club
Pinkham Notch Camp
P. O. Box 298
Gorham, NH 03581-0298
(603) 466-2721
www.outdoors.org
Kinsman Notch, NH, to Grafton Notch, ME

Maine Appalachian Trail Club
P. O. Box 283
Augusta, ME 04332-0283
www.matc.org
Grafton Notch to Katahdin, ME

NON-MAINTAINING A.T. CLUBS

A.T. Club of Florida
c/o Grace Tyner
1310 Quail Drive
Sarasota, FL 34231
(941) 921-1467
gatyner@ix.netcom.com
ATC Supporting Organization

A.T. Club of Alabama
P. O. Box 381842
Birmingham, AL 35238
www.sport.al.com/sport/atca

Lower Appalachian Trail Association
507 Broadway
Sylacauga, AL 35150

Illinois A.T. Club
c/o Norbert Simon
1508 Hinman Avenue, Apt. 4-B
Evanston, IL 60201
(847) 869-9818
nasimon4@attbi.com

International Appalachian Trail
27 Flying Point Road
Freeport, ME 04032
(207) 865-6233
www.internationalat.org

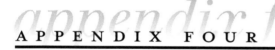

APPENDIX FOUR

The search engine Google turned up 199,000 results for an "Appalachian Trail" search. How do you sort through all the information on the Web? Try the few sites listed below as they provide good sources of information and have links to many more sites.

A.T. and Thru-hiking of Related Interest

The Appalachian Trail Conservancy (**www.appalachiantrail.org**)   The official website for the group that oversees the maintenance and support of the Appalachian Trail.

The Appalachian Trail Homepage (**fred.net/kathy/at.html**)   This unofficial A.T. homepage was the first big Web site devoted to the Appalachian Trail and it stills boasts lots of good information.

Appalachian Long Distance Hikers Association (**www.aldha.org**)

10 Benning Street, PMB 224, West Lebanon, NH 03784

ALDHA holds the annual gathering of long-distance hikers each year to bring together past distance hikers with those dreaming of a future hike. The group also edits the *A.T. Thru-Hiker's Companion,* publishes a newsletter, and sponsors work trips on the A.T.

The Appalachian National Scenic Trail Homepage (**www.nps.gov/appa**)   The National Park Service's official A.T. Web site.

Appalachian Trail Mailing List (**www.backcountry.net**)   Sign on the Appalachian Trail e-mail discussion list at backcountry.net. You can also post a message as a guest or check out the archives at this Web site.

Great Outdoor Recreation Pages' A.T. Info (**www.gorp.com/gorp/resource/us_trail/ appalach.htm**)   A.T.-specific information at the GORP Web site.

TrailJournals.com (**www.trailjournals.com**)   Addicted to reading trail stories? Then this is your Web site, with journals from more than 500 hikers online.

Trailplace.com (**www.trailplace.com**)   This is Dan Bruce's A.T. megasite, with lots of information on the Trail, journal entries, and much more on this group of Web sites all found through Trailplace.

WhiteBlaze.Net (**www.whiteblaze.net**)   This online community of A.T. enthusiasts is a great way to find information and meet fellow hikers.

Educational

Appalachian Tales (**www.appalachiantales.com**)   A Web site designed to help teachers integrate science, literature, art, current events, and history, using the Appalachian Trail as a springboard.

Leave No Trace, Inc. (**www.lnt.org**)   For the ultimate in minimum-impact camping information, head to the source. Leave No Trace is a nonprofit organization created to spread the word about how to preserve the outdoors we love as we hike, camp, and more.

Backpacking Equipment

Backpacker Magazine's Gear Finder (**www.gearfinder.com**)   Gear tips, reviews, and more from *Backpacker* Magazine at this easy-to-use site.

Backpack Gear Test (**www.BackpackGearTest.org**)   Gear reviews by hikers.

Gear Addict (**www.web-dzine.com/gearaddict**)   A backcountry gear megasite.

First-aid Resources

The following companies all offer varying degrees of certification, from Wilderness First Aid to Wilderness EMT. WMI and SOLO offer courses throughout the US; WMI focuses on western states.

Wilderness Medical Associates

189 Dudley Road

Bryant Pond, ME 04219

Information: (800) 945 3633 or **www.wildmed.com**

SOLO (Stonehearth Open Learning Opportunities)

P. O. Box 3150

Conway NH 03818

Information: (603) 447-6711 or **www.soloschools.com**

Wilderness Medical Institute

P. O. Box 9

413 Main St.

Pitkin, CO 81241

Information: (970) 641-3572 or **wmi.nols.edu**

HIKING WITH THE GLOBAL POSITIONING SYSTEM (GPS)

To gather trail information and navigate, a basic GPS unit such as the Garmin Etrex or Magellan Sportrak is a relatively simple and effective tool. Even if you have not used a GPS unit or have limited experience, the basics are easy to master. Prices for a handheld unit range from $100 to $500. Places to purchase units include the Internet, electronics stores, and even large chains such as Wal-Mart.

The primary objectives of a GPS unit are to collect and track data as you walk and to be used as a navigation tool to reach a specific location. The data you collect while hiking can be downloaded later onto a software program such as TopoUSA ($99 for topos of the entire United States) and will overlay the path you walked on top of digitized topo maps. The trail is displayed as you hiked it and may be edited online.

A Global Positioning System (GPS) unit receives data from 24 satellites that orbit the earth. Originally for military use only, the technology is now available for civilian use. When you turn on your GPS unit, it searches the sky and locks onto as many satellites as possible. The unit displays which satellites are available, the strength of the signal, and the location in the sky.

The unit must lock onto at least three satellites in order to accurately fix a moving 2-D position. With three satellites, latitude and longitude are available but not elevation. After locking onto four satellites, the unit is capable of triangulating your east/west, north/south position and altitude. Without WAAS, explained below, the unit is accurate to within 50 feet horizontally and 62 feet vertically. If your GPS unit is WAAS enabled, accuracy increases to 10 feet horizontally and 20 feet vertically.

WAAS stands for Wide Area Augmentation System. There are two WAAS satellites that receive corrective data from ground stations. This corrected data is then broadcast on the same frequency as that of the other GPS satellites.

Using GPS to Gather Trail Data

For most trails, you should be able to maintain a satellite signal lock for the entire hike. Occasionally, though, you will lose the signal. If you look down at the GPS screen and notice a gap in the track (trail) line, the unit has lost the signal but picked it up again. This can be corrected by joining the lines to fill the gap, once the track data is downloaded. Areas you will have problems locking onto signals include hikes next to sheer walls, hikes that meander between tall buildings, and hikes that pass beneath dense tree cover.

In the case of a hike where it is impossible to keep a locked signal, you should turn off the tracking feature and simply plot waypoints whenever the signal appears. Once downloaded onto the topo software, you can draw the trail by connecting waypoints.

Using GPS to Navigate

A GPS unit is capable of leading you to a specific location. Prior to a hike you may want to upload waypoint or map data to your unit. With the target location in view on your screen, the simplest approach is to walk toward the destination. The cursor arrow, which represents the person holding the unit, will travel toward the target as you walk. If you wander off course, it becomes visually obvious as the track begins to veer away from your desired destination

You may also use the unit's GoTo function. Select a waypoint or location from an uploaded map and direct the unit to lead you there. A steering screen guides the user toward the desired target. It will also indicate your bearing, how far you are off course, your speed, and will estimate your time of arrival.

For more advanced users, pinpoint data from a topo map can be entered manually into a GPS unit. The unit will then guide you to that point. This feature requires that you learn how to decipher easting and northing information supplied on topo maps. A good resource for this activity is *GPS Made Easy* by Lawrence Letham.

INDEX

ABOUT THE AUTHORS

Victoria and Frank Logue hiked the entire Appalachian Trail in 1988. They have returned again and again to hike it in its many parts on day and overnight hikes. Frank served on the Appalachian Trail Conservancy Board of Managers. The Logues were also selected as honorary life members of the Appalachian Long-Distance Hikers Association in 2003.

They are the authors of *The Best of The Appalachian Trail: Day Hikes, The Best of the Appalachian Trail: Overnight Hikes,* and the *Appalachian Trail Fun Book,* among other books. Victoria Logue is the author of *Hiking and Backpacking: Essential Skills to Advanced Techniques.*

The Logues live in Georgia, where Frank works as an Episcopal priest while Victoria writes, and they enjoy sharing their love of nature with their daughter, Griffin. The Logues' Web site is at **www.planetanimals.com/logue.**